Series editor
Wilf Yeo
B Med Sci, MB ChB, MD,
MRCP,
Department of
Pharmacology &
Therapeutics,
Royal Hallamshire Hospital,
Sheffield

Faculty advisor
John Spencer
MB ChB, FRC GP
Department of Primary
Health Care,
University of Newcastle
Medical School,
Newcastle-upon-Tyne

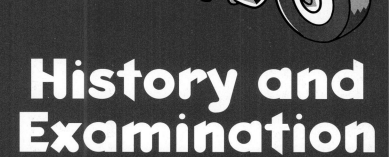

History and Examination

James Marsh
BA, MB BS, MRCP
United Medical and
Dental Schools of Guy's
and St Thomas's
Hospitals (UMDS),
London

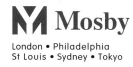 **Mosby**

London • Philadelphia
St Louis • Sydney • Tokyo

Managing Editor	Louise Crowe
Development Editors	Linda Horrell
	and Filipa Maia
Project Manager	Louise Wilson
Designer	Greg Smith
Layout	Mark Howard
Illustration Management	Danny Pyne
Illustrator	Matthew McClements
Cover Design	Greg Smith
Production	Gudrun Hughes
Index	Janine Ross

ISBN 0 7234 3146 9

Copyright © Mosby International Ltd, 1999.

Published by Mosby, an imprint of Mosby International Ltd, Lynton House, 7–12 Tavistock Square, London WC1H 9LB, UK.

Printed by GraphyCems, Navarra, Spain.
Text set in Crash Course–VAG Light; captions in Crash Course–VAG Thin.

Cataloguing in Publication Data
A catalogue records for this book is available from the British Library.

Preface

The clerking is the cornerstone of medical practice. The aim of this book is to guide the student through the daunting task of collecting and restructuring the vast amount of information obtained from taking a history and the examination. The student is encouraged to develop an enquiring approach within a systematic framework so that all important information will be acquired. Following on from this, the student can formulate a clear path towards a differential diagnosis and management plan.

This book is primarily designed as a revision aid for students approaching examinations. The first two sections cover history taking and examination and are divided into body systems. A basic skeleton clerking is presented at the start of each section so that a structured approach can be adopted. Specific examples of different presentations or pathologies are then presented, illustrating how the history or examination can be adapted to different circumstances. The third section helps the student to collate information in the clerking, so that it can be structured and communicated in a digestible form allowing appropriate further investigations and therapeutic strategies to be implemented. Every patient is different – this is part of the challenge of medicine!

James Marsh

In spite of the vast array of technology now available to assist doctors in their work with patients, the role of the history and examination remains central in both diagnosis and management. A quarter of a century ago George Engel said '...the interview is potentially the most powerful, sensitive instrument at the command of the physician'. The move towards a more patient-centred clinical method in recent years has, if anything, increased the importance of the history and examination. The benefits of good communication go beyond making an accurate diagnosis – concordance with treatment is more likely, patient outcomes are improved, doctors feel more satisfied with their work, and complaints and litigation are reduced. Similarly, the physical examination does more than to help confirm your clinical hunches. It also enables you to make a more discriminating use of diagnostic technology, something that demonstrates a professional approach to the patient and will be appreciated by both your patients and the public purse.

This book offers a comprehensive, user-friendly guide to history-taking and physical examination. A flexible and discriminating approach is encouraged, one that is sensitive to patients' ideas, concerns and expectations. I am sure *Crash Course: History and Examination* will be useful to you not only in passing your exams, but beyond the dreaded long and short cases into 'real life'. James Marsh is to be congratulated for his efforts in authoring this text.

John Spencer
Faculty Advisor

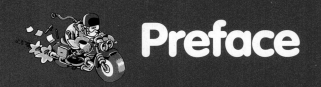

Preface

So you have an exam in medicine and you don't know where to start? The answer is easy – start with *Crash Course*. Medicine is fun to learn if you can bring it to life with patients who need their problems solving. This series of books does just that, focusing on learning methods to find the right path through the differential diagnosis, and offering treatment promptly.

The *Crash Course* Series is designed to help you in preparing for exams and includes informative diagrams and Hint and Tip boxes to help you remember concepts. The books are comprehensive, accurate and well balanced, and should enable you to learn each subject well. To check that you did learn something from the book, (rather than just flashing it in front of your eyes!), we have added a self-assessment section in the usual format of most medical exams – multiple-choice and short-answer questions (with answers), and case studies for self-directed learning. Good luck!

Wilf Yeo
Series Editor (Clinical Sciences)

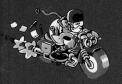# Acknowledgements

With thanks to Christopher Chan for his involvement in the early stages of this book.

Figure Credits

Figures 5.1, 5.2, 5.12, 14.6, 14.7, 14.12, 14.13, 14.15, 14.19 and 20.14 taken from *Clinical Examination 2e* by O. Epstein, G.D. Perkin, D.P. de Bono and J. Cookson. TMIP, 1997.

Figures 7.9, 16.5, 16.7, 16.13, 16.14, 16.16, 16.20, 16.25 and 21.1 from *Crash Course: Nervous System and Special Senses* by D. Lasserson, C. Gabriel and B. Sharrack. Mosby International, 1998.

Figures 15.5 and 15.6 from *Crash Course: Endocrine and Reproductive Systems* by M. Debuse, Mosby International, 1998.

Figure 20.4 from *Crash Course: Musculoskeletal System* by S. Biswas and R. Iqbal. Mosby International, 1998.

Figure 23.1A from *A Color Atlas of Clinical Medicine 2e* by C.D. Forbes and W.F. Jackson. TMIP, 1997.

Contents

Contents

To Jane

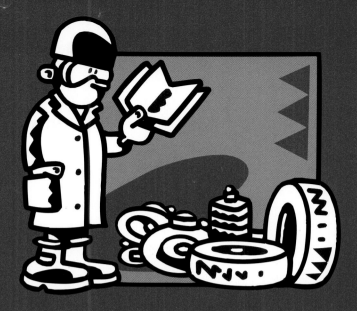

HISTORY

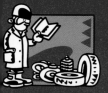

1. Introduction to History Taking

BASIC PRINCIPLES

The principal aims of medical clerking are to establish:
- What is wrong with the patient?
- How do these problems impact on the patient's life?

The standard approach is to obtain the history before conducting a physical examination and requesting appropriate investigations. Despite being discussed as separate chapters, these components of the clerking interlock with each other in a dynamic fashion from the moment that the doctor meets the patient.

The medical history has a traditional format, but it should not be considered as a rigid interrogation and checklist of questions. Although a structured approach is needed, it is important to adopt a flexible attitude, adapting your questions and differential diagnosis as information is received. The process of formulating a differential diagnosis starts as soon as the patient describes his or her presenting complaint. The symptom should be explored in detail so that possible diagnoses can be excluded, others can be introduced, and the relative probability of each assessed. Once the patient has described his or her main symptoms, specific questions should be asked to refine the differential diagnosis. Thus the process of history taking is an active skill, and not one of passive listening.

OBTAINING AND ASSESSING INFORMATION

Gleaning the important information is a fine art and takes years to master. Every medical student has experienced the frustration of taking a garbled, incoherent history from a rambling patient, only to see a consultant ask one or two seemingly simple questions that make the underlying diagnosis become embarrassingly straightforward.

The traditional approach is to start by asking 'open' questions, for example:
- "Tell me about your pain!"
- "Why have you come to hospital today?"

This gives patients the opportunity to tell you how they perceive their problems before the agenda is taken out of their hands, and your own prejudices take over. (It is surprising how often the doctor and patient focus on different problems.) By careful steering and gentle coaxing, even the most garrulous patients can usually give full, clear, and reasonably concise descriptions of their current symptoms. It is also necessary to ask 'closed' questions for further clarification, for example:
- "Does your abdominal pain get worse after eating?"
- "Did you black out completely or just feel lightheaded?"

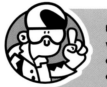

It is a matter of judgement when to start interrupting and asking closed questions, but as a general rule, think twice before interrupting a patient in full flow. If specific questions are introduced too early, vital information may never come to light.

It is also important to obtain information on the impact the patients' illness has, not only physically but also in a wider context, psychologically and socially. A given pathological process affects individuals in very different ways, depending upon factors such as lifestyle, social circumstances, attitude to illness, and other medical problems. This information is vital for a full assessment and also reassures patients that the doctor is taking a genuine interest in them and not just their chest pain, arthritis, etc. Information to explore includes:
- Ideas. What does the patient think is wrong?
- Concerns. What is the patient worried might be wrong?
- Expectations. What does the patient think is going to happen in the consultation and regarding his or her future health? What might happen following the consultation? (e.g. investigations, operations).

RELATIONSHIP WITH THE PATIENT

The atmosphere and setting is important when taking a history. Patients should feel free to express their fears and concerns without fear or embarrassment. An absolute air of confidentiality should be tacitly created. At the same time, take note of any non-verbal signs (e.g. hostility, embarrassment). Often the most crucial information needs to be coaxed out of the patient. Never appear to be in a rush. Patients expect and deserve full attention and sympathy for their problems. It is not unusual for patients to express their real concerns just as they are leaving the consulting room.

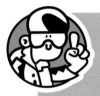

However tempting, do not ignore throwaway comments from the patient. They often carry the key to the whole problem. Never be in a rush. Time invested in taking a good history pays dividends in the long term.

It is often useful (even if potentially time-consuming), to ask patients at the end of a consultation if there is anything else they wish to discuss. If patients feel at ease with you, they will talk more freely. They should feel confident not only in your diagnostic abilities, but also in your empathy, understanding, and motivation. After all, you are acting as their advocate. This process should start as soon as you greet patients.

Remember that first impressions really do matter. Appear friendly, but professional. Patients must have confidence in your abilities to act on their behalf.

DIFFICULT CONSULTATIONS

In certain circumstances the history can be considerably more difficult to obtain, for example if:
- There is a language barrier.
- The patient is confused, hostile, or unconscious.

There is, however, rarely any justification for resorting to a veterinary approach. Remember that the history is the most important part of the clerking. If there is a language barrier, help the patient to relax, do not rush, explain everything clearly, and if necessary obtain an interpreter. If the patient is confused or unconscious, history taking is still vital. A relative, carer, nursing home worker, or other witness is usually available to provide information. This process is time consuming, but worthwhile. Most doctors have learned from bitter experience!

The history is the most important part of the patient's assessment as it provides 80% of the information required to make a diagnosis.

OVERVIEW OF HISTORY SECTION

The first section of this book focuses on the history. Chapter 2 outlines the basic structure of a medical history, detailing the bare skeleton of the history. It is important to adopt a systematic approach so that all relevant information is obtained. The following chapters are used to illustrate the need to be flexible within that basic format, adapting your questions to different circumstances, so that differential diagnoses can be explored. The examples of medical histories are not intended to provide a rigid checklist of questions. History taking is a highly individual skill, and students will need to adopt their own style. The examples provided are only a framework, and should be adapted to suit your own preferences and the individual patient.

2. The History

INTRODUCTORY STATEMENT

Before taking a detailed history it is essential to obtain some background information from the patient. This should include the patient's:
- Name.
- Age.
- Sex.
- Occupation.
- Presenting complaint.

Ideally, try to use the words that the patient has used (e.g. people rarely complain of 'dyspnoea', but will say that they feel 'short of breath'). This statement should be short and pithy, for example "John Smith is a 56-year-old electrician complaining of chest pain".

This information is vital as it helps you (and any listeners) focus interest during the course of the subsequent history, so that appropriate questions can be anticipated if the patient does not volunteer the information. The process of forming a differential diagnosis should have already begun, but at this stage, it will by necessity be broad.

HISTORY OF PRESENTING COMPLAINT

This is the main component of the history. A detailed, thorough investigation into the current illness is performed. This is usually composed of two sequential (but often overlapping) stages:
- The patient's account of the symptoms.
- Specific, detailed questions by the doctor.

The relative proportion of each component depends upon the underlying problem, the communication skills of the patient, and the often underestimated listening skills of the doctor. Listening should be an active process. Ideally, the patient should be given every opportunity to talk freely at the start of the consultation with minimal interruption. A common mistake made by most students (and doctors) is to intervene too early.

Patients must feel that they are getting a fair hearing and have had an adequate opportunity to express themselves. They should be made to feel that the doctor is listening carefully and has a genuine concern for their problems. Subtle nuances are often missed if the doctor seizes the agenda too early.

A combination of art, experience, and patience determines when and how to interrupt a patient in full flow. It is prudent to allow the patient to drift a little (especially if you are inexperienced at taking histories). Make a mental note of the most important features of the narrative and issues that require clarification.

The full circumstances surrounding a single event or symptom need to be explored in a systematic manner so that a complete mental image can be obtained.

An example of this approach is illustrated below.

A patient complains of pain
Explore in detail the circumstances surrounding the episode so that a complete picture can be obtained.

What was the patient doing immediately before the episode?
Ascertain exactly what the patient was doing at the time of the onset of the pain (e.g. running, arguing with partner, sitting in chair).

Speed of onset
Determine the rate of development of pain (e.g. seconds, minutes, hours, days). It may be helpful to draw a graph of symptoms versus time (Figs 2.1 and 2.2).

Time of onset
Try to obtain exact times and dates if appropriate.

Subsequent time course
Map out the fluctuations in symptoms with time.

Duration
How long did the pain last? Patients often overestimate the duration of symptoms.

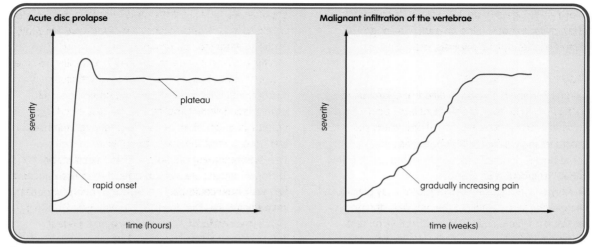

Fig. 2.1 The typical time course of two different types of back pain, which are of the same severity at presentation but of different aetiology.

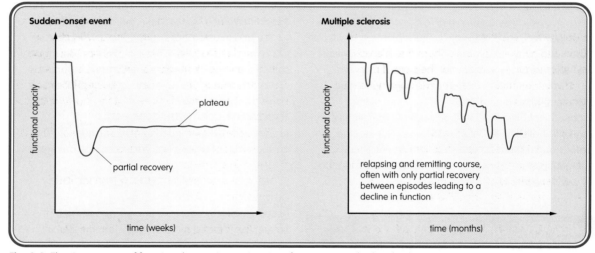

Fig. 2.2 The time course of functional capacity against time for a patient who has had a stroke or has multiple sclerosis. It is important to consider not only the speed of onset of a particular symptom, but its subsequent time course.

Nature of pain

It is particularly useful to record direct quotations from the patient such as:

- "Like a stabbing knife".
- "Like being compressed by a vice".

They are often very descriptive and reflect how a particular symptom is affecting the patient rather than the doctor's interpretation. Many patients are less colourful in their language and may need help to describe a symptom. You could then provide examples such as: "Would you describe the pain as burning, stabbing, crushing, throbbing, or something else?"

Radiation

Radiation of pain is important and often gives clues to the aetiology. For example, the pain of a prolapsed intervertebral disc usually radiates down the back of one leg whereas muscular strain is usually well localized.

Associated symptoms

Pain rarely occurs in isolation. Associated symptoms are often characteristic of certain pathological processes. For example, if a patient describes pleuritic chest pain, ask about the presence of cough, dyspnoea, fever, haemoptysis, etc.

Aggravating features
Different types of pain have different aggravating factors. For example, mechanical back pain is often exacerbated by exercise, but inflammatory pain may be worse after a period of prolonged rest.

Relieving factors
Factors producing relief of symptoms may give clues to the aetiology or severity of the pain (e.g. the pain of intermittent claudication resolves rapidly on rest compared with the pain of critical limb ischaemia).

Recovery
Note the time and speed of recovery.

Residual symptoms
Once the pain has resolved, there are often ongoing symptoms: for example, after the pain of myocardial infarction the patient often reports ongoing fatigue, dyspnoea, or palpitations.

Effect of any interventions
Ask about the effect of interventions, for example:
- "Did your chest pain get any better after taking a glyceryl trinitrate (GTN) tablet?"
- "Did the pain go when you stopped running?"

In the event of repeated symptoms additional information is also needed, for example frequency and pattern (e.g. getting progressively better or worse, more or less easily provoked).

Previous episodes
Ask the patient if he or she has had a similar episode of pain before.

Interpreting information
Do not accept the patient's (or the doctor's) interpretation of symptoms at face value. At this stage, you are most interested in what the patient was 'actually' experiencing. If the patient has been given a label for the symptoms, it may be helpful to know by whom, and on what evidence. For example, if the patient says "My doctor tells me I have angina!", find

out whether the patient has had investigations such as an exercise test, angiography, or electrocardiography, and if so what the results were.

Often different patients mean different things by the same phrase. Be wary! For example, dizziness may relate to vertigo, pre-syncope, muzziness, etc. This clearly has different implications for the underlying diagnosis. In addition, try to make your questions as clear and unambiguous as possible.

When recording the history try to keep it as brief and 'punchy' as possible. An example of a history obtained for chest pain could be: "He describes a sudden-onset retrosternal chest tightness 'like a tight band' radiating to the jaw and left arm every time he climbs the staircase from the underground station (approximately 100 steps). He has a sensation that he needs to stop and rest immediately, and also feels mildly nauseated, short of breath, and occasionally sweaty. He never has palpitations, lightheadedness, nor syncopal episodes. The pain is relieved within two minutes of resting or seconds after placing a GTN tablet under his tongue, and he can then continue his daily activities. He has noticed that on a cold or windy day, the pain comes on earlier, but otherwise has been stable over the past two months".

This illustrates the need to play an active role in the discussion, being always aware of:
- The differential diagnosis.
- How the symptoms interfere with functional activities.

Wherever possible, try to quantify the symptoms objectively. In addition, the presence of relevant 'negative' symptoms creates a more complete picture.

A long list of 'negatives' is very dull and judgement is needed when deciding which ones to include in the narrative. This is where experience helps when presenting the history. Try to imagine yourself as the listener, and consider carefully what information you would want to know.

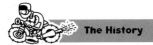

Rounding off the history

By asking patients what they think the cause of their symptoms might be, an interesting insight is always provided. They are often worried about the consequences of what appears to be a trivial symptom to an objective observer. It is impossible to offer appropriate reassurance or counselling without this knowledge. Furthermore, if the patient's own judgement differs significantly from the doctor's, the doctor must reassess how he or she arrived at the differential diagnosis.

Often, a history is very complicated, or the patient appears to have given a contradictory account. It is helpful to read back your recollection of the history to the patient so that he or she can verify its accuracy—you will have opportunity to place your own interpretation at a later stage! You should both be in agreement about the facts before you introduce your own bias! It provides a message to the patient that you have been listening to his or her concerns. This is a useful way of focusing patients, especially if they are rambling. Finally, it is a good way of ending the history.

 It is helpful to clarify your interpretaion of the history by reading back your notes to the patient

Summary

When taking the history of the presenting complaint, remember the following:

- The primary objective is to obtain a comprehensive but succinct account of the presenting symptom(s).
- Allow patients sufficient opportunity to describe their symptoms at the start.
- Resist the temptation to interrupt too early and too frequently.
- If patients drift, gently coax and steer them back on course to the main focus.
- Ask specific questions to clarify, obtain more detail, or to investigate potential diagnoses only after the patient has described his or her symptoms,.
- Sometimes negative answers are more important than positive answers.
- Ask patients what they think may be causing the symptoms.

- If the history is complicated, recount your interpretation of events back to the patient to ensure that your versions are concordant.
- Attempt to be as systematic and objective as possible. Look for collateral evidence to support any statement, especially if it is related to someone's interpretation of symptoms.
- Ask easily understood, unambiguous questions.
- If the patient presents with more than one complaint this process may need repeating for each complaint.

PAST MEDICAL HISTORY

This is important for placing the current illness in the context of past events, which are often related. A review of the past medical history should include the points addressed below.

Previous hospital admissions

Outline essential information, such as:

- Diagnoses/problems.
- Dates and places.
- Treatment and investigations.

Occasionally, verification of previous events may be necessary, particularly if the patient has had a complicated hospital admission. This may prevent repetition of unnecessary (and sometimes harmful) investigations. The patient's recollection may be hazy, especially of events occurring within hospital (e.g. investigations for acute renal failure).

Operations

List procedures chronologically in a similar way to that described above for hospital admissions.

Known medical or psychiatric conditions

Remember to have a healthy scepticism about labels given to the patient. If necessary, explore how a diagnosis has been established.

Problems related to underlying present illness

Ask about particular risk factors or associated diseases related to the primary complaint. For example, if a patient presents with chest pain, ask specifically about:

- Previous episodes of angina and myocardial infarction.
- Strokes and transient ischaemic attacks (TIAs).
- Diabetes mellitus.
- Hypertension.
- Hypercholesterolaemia.

This is the component of the past medical history that takes the most skill. An awareness of the likely differential diagnosis is needed. Remember that the history should be adapted to different circumstances. Listening should be active, and relevant negative information often provides as much information as positive facts.

DRUG HISTORY

A complete list of current medication with doses is a minimum requirement. Very often, more detailed information is needed.

Why is drug history important?

A detailed drug history is important because:

- It may give an indication of disease processes that the patient was either unaware of or has failed to mention (e.g. thyroxine suggestive of hypothyroidism, amiodarone suggestive of arrhythmia).
- The drugs may be the cause of the present symptoms due to adverse effects or drug interactions (e.g. headache induced by nitrates used to treat angina, dyspnoea and lethargy induced by β-blockers). Try to establish a temporal relationship between the initiation or change of medication and the onset of new symptoms.
- Conversely, withdrawal of therapy may be responsible for the current symptoms (e.g. withdrawal of diuretics may lead to swollen ankles and orthopnoea; withdrawal of β-blockers may result in chest pain and palpitations).
- It provides an opportunity to explore the patient's understanding of the disease, often highlighting a need for further education (e.g. the controlled use and technique of inhaling glucocorticosteroids and bronchodilators by the asthmatic patient).
- The potential therapeutic options for the presenting illness can be explored.

Often, even more detail of distant therapy is needed (e.g. second-line therapy for rheumatoid arthritis, Fig. 2.3). This is particularly important when the therapeutic options are limited or if the agents used are potentially toxic (e.g. chemotherapy for malignancy, immunosuppresssive agents for nephrotic syndrome).

Check compliance and explore the reasons for non-compliance, such as:

- Intolerable side effects.
- Perceived lack of efficacy.
- Ignorance.
- Poor communication from prescribing physician.
- Four times daily medication instead of once daily.

This exploration of compliance must be done very sensitively in an effort not to appear to be judgemental. Patients do not like admitting that they have not taken medication prescribed on their behalf. Use statements such as "Do you ever have difficulty taking your tablets?" or "Do you ever forget to take your tablets?" Even when approached sensitively, few patients admit poor compliance. This is important because there is no point in inexorably increasing the dose of medication if it is not being taken. Common culprits include antihypertensive agents.

Example of drug history for a patient with rheumatoid arthritis			
Drug	**Dates**	**Efficacy**	**Reason for discontinuation**
gold	Jan. 92–Jun. 93	progressive erosions	lack of effect; proteinuria 1 g/24 h
penicillamine	Jun. 93–Feb. 94	remission; no progressive erosions, no flares	rash
methotrexate	Feb. 94–Jun. 96	good response	hepatotoxicity (fibrosis on biopsy)
azathioprine	Jun. 96–ongoing	in remission	

Fig. 2.3 Example of drug history for a patient with rheumatoid arthritis.

Ask specifically about use of over-the-counter (OTC) medication, herbal remedies, and (in women) oral contraceptives. These are often not considered to be 'medication'. Associated problems, however, include analgesic nephropathy with many simple analgesic agents and hepatic veno-occlusive disease with 'bush tea'.

In the unconscious patient, check for the use of agents whose use or abrupt withdrawal may have contributed to coma. For example, glucocorticosteroids, anticoagulants, anti-epileptics, and insulin. The patient may carry a card detailing this information or wear a 'medicalert' bracelet.

Ask to see the patient's medicines. This provides extra insight into the patient's understanding as well as compliance.

HISTORY OF DRUG ALLERGY

This follows naturally from the drug history. As with other sections of the history, a systematic approach is rewarded.

Many people think that they have an allergy to medication, but a healthy scepticism is needed when assessing this. Always enquire how the 'allergy' was manifested, for example 'stomach upset' after the use of antibiotics is common, and very rarely an allergic phenomenon. Skin rashes are much more likely to represent a true allergy.

It is important to clarify the circumstances of a suspected allergic reaction. Attempt to establish a 'temporal relationship' between the drug administration and the allergic manifestation. For example, it is not uncommon for a rash to be part of a viral illness or for a rash to be an epiphenomenon—patients with glandular fever who are prescribed amoxycillin will develop a macular erythematous rash. This is not an allergic phenomenon.

Enquire whether the patient has ever been 'rechallenged' with the same drug, and if so whether any reaction occurred. However, in most cases of uncertainty, it is usually safest to assume that the patient does have an allergy, and to avoid the suspected drug.

Finally, enquire about the presence of atopic conditions (e.g. eczema, hay fever, asthma, urticaria, etc.).

SOCIAL HISTORY

The social history is crucial for every patient as it provides information on how the disease and patient interact at a functional level. It is particularly important that it is detailed in elderly, frail, or socially isolated patients. Try to obtain a picture of daily activities, and consider the impact of the disease at each stage.

An example is presented below.

An elderly person presents with a hemiplegia
What is the structure of the home?
Consider the physical characteristics of the home as this will affect mobility and ability to function independently, for example:
- Is it a flat or a house?
- If it is a flat, what floor is it on and is there a lift?
- How many bedrooms are there?
- What access is there to the house, bedroom, kitchen, toilet, etc. (e.g. stairs, ramps)?

Who are the potential carers?
Enquire about the structure of the household and whether other members of the household are in the house during the day and physically fit. Find out whether any family members live nearby. Are there any other potential local carers?

Can the patient perform the usual activities of daily living?
Assess the practicalities of routine activities such as:
- Getting in and out of bed.
- Dressing.
- Toileting (mobility and continence).
- Cooking and eating.
- Bathing.
- Shopping.

What level of social support is already provided for the patient?
The patient may already be known to the social services. Enquire specifically about district nursing, meals on wheels, home help, social worker, etc.

Other patients may require the help of occupational therapists (e.g. patients with rheumatoid arthritis may need assessment for aids for eating, ramps for access to the home, stair rails, stair lifts, bath seats, etc.).

The young patient

Younger patients present different problems and an illness may interfere with their lifestyle or be a direct result of it. It is important to find out the following information.

Occupation

Consider whether the occupation may have predisposed to the current illness, for example:

- Asbestos exposure in dockyard workers, boiler makers.
- Pneumoconiosis in coal miners.
- Non-specific chest pain in people presenting with stress.

Consider whether the present illness may interfere with the ability to continue with the patient's occupation, for example:

- Epilepsy or myocardial infarction in the driver of a heavy goods vehicle.
- Ischaemic heart disease or rheumatoid arthritis in a manual worker.

Do not forget that lack of employment may contribute to the presenting illness. There is a well-documented association with the onset of morbidity (both physical and psychological) and unemployment.

If the patient is seeking a certificate for prolonged absence from work, the home and work circumstances clearly need to be explored in detail.

Hobbies

These may be the cause of the illness (e.g. pigeon-fancier's lung) or be precluded by the current illness (e.g. squash if the patient has newly diagnosed angina).

Travel

World travel is increasingly common and it is therefore important to be aware of recent travel, for example consider:

- Malaria in a patient who has returned from an endemic area and presents with fever.
- Hepatitis A in a person with jaundice who has been to an endemic area.
- Schistosomiasis in a patient presenting with haematuria.

Other sources of stress

Common causes include financial difficulties, job insecurity, or strained relationships at home. The list, however, is endless and recognition depends upon great sensitivity by the doctor.

Recreational drugs

It is often appropriate to enquire specifically about the use of recreational drugs, for example:

- If immunodeficiency is suspected.
- Needle marks are spotted.
- The patient presents with a decreased level of consciousness.

Risk factors for human immunodeficiency virus (HIV) and hepatitis B

These diseases are becoming more common and an increasing index of suspicion is needed, especially for those patients with risk factors, for example:

- Haemophiliacs.
- Recipients of blood transfusion in Africa since 1977.
- Sexual partners of prostitutes.
- Intravenous drug users.
- Sexually active homosexuals.
- Individuals with multiple sexual partners partaking in unprotected sexual intercourse.
- Sexual partners of the above groups.

Smoking

It is obligatory to ask every patient about cigarette smoking. A useful concept is 'pack years' (i.e. the number of packs of cigarettes smoked daily multiplied by the years of smoking). Do not forget other forms of smoking.

Alcohol

Alcohol plays a contributory role in many illnesses. An attempt should be made to estimate consumption for every patient. This is usually quoted in units/week. One unit equals:

- 1/2 pint of beer.
- 1 glass of wine.
- 1 single measure of spirit.

In certain circumstances, a more detailed history is appropriate. It is sometimes helpful to work through a typical drinking day for someone you suspect is a heavy drinker. Remember that, because patients believe that doctors are likely to disapprove of heavy drinking, denial is common. At this stage in the consultation it is not your job to be judgemental!

A useful screening questionnaire is the CAGE test:

- **C**: Have you ever felt you ought to CUT down on your drinking?
- **A**: Has anyone ANNOYED you by criticising your drinking?
- **G**: Have you ever felt GUILTY about your drinking?
- **E**: Have you ever had a drink first thing in the morning to steady your nerves or to get rid of a hangover (EYE opener)?

Nutrition

An attempt should be made to assess nutritional status. A detailed history is needed for certain patients (e.g. those presenting with weight loss or iron-, folate-, or vitamin B_{12}-deficiency anaemia).

FAMILY HISTORY

Information about the health and age of other family members is often instructive, particularly for young patients or those with a suspected inherited disease. It is helpful to draw a family tree (Fig. 2.4).

Some diseases have a predictable mode of inheritance (Figs 2.5 and 2.6), for example:

- Autosomal dominant (e.g. Huntington's chorea, adult polycystic kidneys).
- Autosomal recessive (e.g. cystic fibrosis).
- X-linked dominant (e.g. vitamin D-resistant rickets).
- X-linked recessive (e.g. colour blindness).

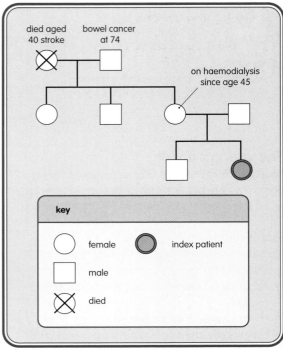

Fig. 2.4 A typical family tree written in hospital notes demonstrating family members affected by autosomal dominant polycystic kidneys.

Other disorders do not have a mendelian mode of inheritance, but there is often a discernible genetic component, and family history is still significant. Such disorders include:

- Hypertension.
- Ischaemic heart disease.
- Schizophrenia.
- Breast cancer.

Even if the suspected disease has no recognized inheritable factor, it is useful to record a family tree with causes of death or major diseases. Doing this with the patient may open the door to some of the patient's concerns and may provide a useful insight into relationships within the family.

In some circumstances, a particularly high level of suspicion is needed, for example the young child with epileptic fits or the young boy with deafness and haematuria due to Alport's syndrome.

A detailed family history may help to stratify risk factors in order to aid diagnosis or counselling asymptomatic relatives.

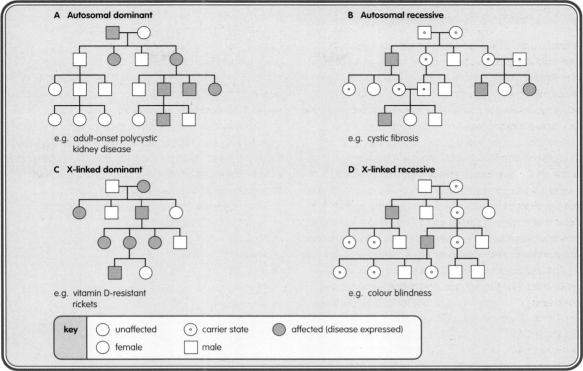

Fig. 2.5 Different modes of Mendelian inheritance. (A) The phenotype is expressed in each generation. On average, 50% of the offspring of an affected individual will have the characteristic. Males and females are equally affected. (B) Only 25% of the offspring of a couple carrying the gene will be affected. Males and females have the characteristic with equal frequency. These diseases are much more common in highly inbred populations, especially if there is consanguinous marriage. (C) All of the female offspring of an affected male will be affected, while 50% of the male offspring of an affected female will also be affected. (D) The phenotype is not expressed in females (except for the very rare homozygous state), while 50% of the female offspring of a carrier will be carriers, and 50% of the male offspring will show the characteristic.

Fig. 2.6 Examples of some inherited disorders.

Examples of some inherited disorders	
Pattern of inheritance	**Examples**
autosomal dominant	adult-onset polycystic kidney disease; achondroplasia; neurofibromatosis; hereditary spherocytosis; familial adenomatous polyposis; tuberous sclerosis
autosomal recessive	cystic fibrosis; Gaucher's disease; sickle-cell anaemia; infantile polycystic kidney disease;
X-linked recessive	colour blindness; haemophilia A; Christmas disease
X-linked dominant	vitamin D-resistant rickets

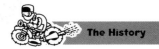
REVIEW OF SYMPTOMS

A brief review of symptoms in a systems enquiry is essential in a detailed history. It may suggest other disorders that have not been considered or highlight potentially serious complications that a patient may have considered to be trivial. In addition, it may be used as a screening process to highlight aspects of the history that require more detailed attention.

With practice, it is possible to cover this aspect of the history in a few minutes and is time well invested.

It is helpful to consider this section in systems. When the presenting complaint appears to relate to one system, this system should be promoted to the detailed history of the presenting complaint, and a more detailed enquiry performed. The absence of particular symptoms attains a greater significance: for example when a patient describes chest pain, the presence or absence of dyspnoea or palpitations is clearly more relevant than when the presenting complaint is headache.

The systems enquiry is often the most difficult component of the history to interpret. The significance of each symptom and its relevance to the primary complaint needs to be analysed. This may lead to a review of the differential diagnosis and new questions to either confirm or refute new suspicions.

With a little practice, it is possible to draw up your own list of questions that can be asked and answered rapidly. It is helpful to consider each system of the body in turn. Some important symptoms and associated screening questions are listed in Figs 2.7–2.11.

Other general symptoms to consider include:
- Early morning stiffness.
- Mobility.
- Fevers.
- Sweats.
- Weight loss.
- Tiredness.

Some screening questions for the cardiovascular system in the review of symptoms	
Symptom	**Questions**
chest pain	explore in detail; in particular note the characteristic of the pain (e.g. cardiac, musculoskeletal, pleuritic, pericarditic, oesophageal, etc.)
dyspnoea	quantify exercise tolerance; ascertain whether predominant pathology is cardiovascular or respiratory
orthopnoea	quantify number of pillows needed ("what would happen if you were forced to sleep with no pillows?"); enquire specifically about paroxysmal nocturnal dyspnoea ("do you ever wake up in the night gasping for breath and need to sit on the side of your bed?")
ankle swelling	duration; degree; presence of facial or genital oedema, ascites
fatigue	"when did you last feel completely well?"; "if I asked you to walk to the train station, what would make you stop?" (e.g. dyspnoea, chest pain, claudication, fatigue, etc.)

Fig. 2.7 Some screening questions for the cardiovascular system in the review of symptoms.

Some screening questions for the respiratory system in the review of symptoms	
Symptom	**Questions**
dyspnoea	see Fig. 2.7
cough	duration; sputum production; constitutional symptoms (e.g. coryza, fever, malaise, weight loss); time of day (e.g. left heart failure or asthma may present with night-time cough)
sputum production	amount per day (e.g. teaspoonful, eggcupful, etc.); characteristics (colour, tenacity, etc.); foul taste (e.g. anaerobic infection); associated haemoptysis, chest pain
wheeze	provoking factors (e.g. exercise, cold weather, house dust, etc.)

Fig. 2.8 Some screening questions for the respiratory system in the review of symptoms.

Some screening questions for the gastrointestinal system in the review of symptoms	
Symptom	**Questions**
weight loss	"is your loss in weight intentional?"; quantify; appetite; constitutional symptoms (e.g. fever, malaise, fatigue, etc); diarrhoea, vomiting
nausea, vomiting	duration, frequency; time of day (e.g. early morning symptoms may indicate raised intracranial pressure); obvious precipitating factors (e.g. drugs, alcohol, pregnancy, food poisoning); presence of haemoptysis
dysphagia	"where does the food appear to get stuck?"
abdominal pain	needs to be explored in detail; establish site, acute versus chronic; characteristics; relationship to food; indigestion; relieving factors, etc.
stool frequency	remember that different people have very different perceptions about the terms 'constipation' and 'diarrhoea'; establish the patient's usual bowel habit and what changes have occurred for both frequency and stool consistency; rectal bleeding; duration of symptoms

Fig. 2.9 Some screening questions for the gastrointestinal system in the review of symptoms.

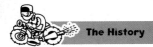

Some screening questions for the genitourinary system in the review of symptoms	
Symptom	**Questions**
urinary frequency	if abnormal, quantify the number of times that urine is passed during the day and night (e.g. day/night = 6–8/2)
poor stream dysuria	enquire about other features of prostatism (nocturia, hesitancy, terminal dribbling, etc.)
haematuria	timing during the urinary stream; constitutional symptoms; urinary frequency; appearance of urine (e.g. cloudy, blood, offensive smell); degree of blood (e.g. clots, 'like claret', bloodstained, etc.)
menstruation	cycle length, duration of menstruation, pain, menorrhagia, etc.
sexual activity	many patients are not willing to discuss their sexual history and often it is not relevant; relevant questions may cover number of sexual partners, "do you practise safe sex?", homosexual encounters, libido, impotence, etc.

Fig. 2.10 Some screening questions for the genitourinary system in the review of symptoms.

Some screening questions for the nervous system	
Symptom	**Questions**
headache	explore features in depth including frequency, nature and location of pain, associated symptoms, timing during day, etc.
blackouts	if the patient describes a blackout, it is essential to devote time to exploring the event as this warrants investigation in its own right, regardless of other symptoms
fits	is the patient a known epileptic?; frequency and control, type of fits, duration of epilepsy, etc.
muscle weakness	duration, pattern of weakness, precipitating events
paraesthesia	distribution (e.g. dermatome, peripheral nerve, etc.).
change in vision	speed of onset. clarify visual acuity (e.g. "can you read newspapers, watch television?" etc.); diplopia
dizziness	clarify exactly what the patient means by dizziness (e.g. vertigo, lightheadedness, muzzy feeling, etc.)

Fig. 2.11 Some screening questions for the nervous system in the review of symptoms.

SUMMARY

At the end of the history it is useful to provide a short summary of two or three sentences encompassing the most salient features. This will help you and the listener focus on the most relevant parts of the ensuing examination.

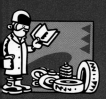

3. Presenting Problems: Cardiovascular System

CHEST PAIN (CARDIAC)

Detailed history
Obtain a detailed account of the pain in a systematic manner as described in Chapter 2, asking specifically about the features discussed below.

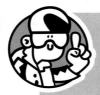

Patients may express the nature of their pain non-verbally — typically by clenching their fist over the sternal region.

Site
Ask patients to indicate on themselves where exactly they experience the pain. The pain is typically retrosternal, but may only be present in the neck, throat, or arms (especially left arm) (Fig. 3.1).

Radiation
The pain may not radiate, but classically goes to the throat and left arm (see Fig. 3.1).

Nature of pain
It is helpful to write down the exact words used by the patient. Cardiac chest pain is usually described as 'tight', 'crushing', 'gripping', 'like a band across my chest', 'a dull ache'. Patients often have difficulty finding words to describe abstract sensations such as pain, but it is important to try to ascertain its nature. You could give alternatives, for example "Would you describe the pain as burning, stabbing, tightness, tearing sensation, or something else?". Remember to try to avoid leading the patient too much!

Often patients have had angina for a long time and may describe a pain as "like my angina, only worse" when experiencing a myocardial infarction.

Make an attempt to distinguish the pain from other types of chest pain (Fig. 3.2). The main types of pain are:
- Cardiac.
- Pleuritic—sharp, stabbing, aggravated by coughing, deep breathing, or occasionally posture.
- Gastrointestinal—often related to food ingestion, may be vague in character or described as burning, may be associated with an acid taste in the mouth.

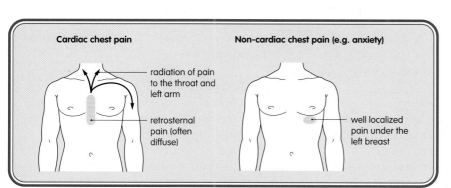

Fig. 3.1 Typical location of cardiac chest pain and non-specific chest pain in an anxious patient. A quick sketch in the notes is often more informative than a long explanation.

Cardiac chest pain
Non-cardiac chest pain (e.g. anxiety)
radiation of pain to the throat and left arm
retrosternal pain (often diffuse)
well localized pain under the left breast

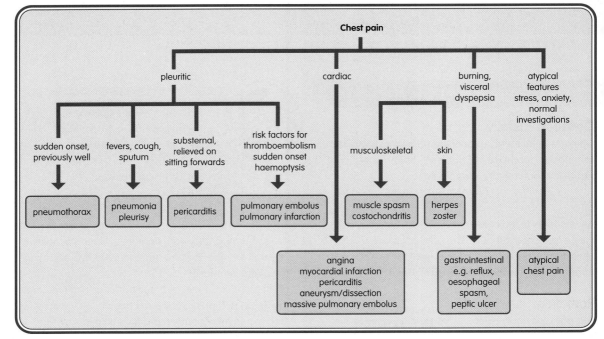

Fig. 3.2 Differential diagnosis of chest pain.

- Musculoskeletal—usually easily recognized; the pain has a superficial quality and is often exaggerated by movement; there is often a good mechanical explanation.
- Atypical—diagnosis is partly by exclusion, partly by its atypical characteristics.

Precipitating factors

Angina is typically provoked by exertion. If the pain is reproducible, try to find out the level of exertion necessary to induce it (e.g. walking up one flight of stairs, 200 metres on the flat). Note if this level of exertion has changed recently. Ask specifically about other precipitating causes (e.g. stress, excitement, sexual intercourse, meals).

If this is the first episode of pain or its nature has changed, it is important to know what the patient was doing 'immediately' before the onset of pain (e.g. stable angina is provoked by a predictable stress, but a myocardial infarction often occurs at rest).

Time course and relieving factors

Angina usually lasts for only a few minutes and is typically relieved by rest. Patients often describe an urge to slow down or stop if they are walking at the onset of pain. Ask the patient exactly how long the pain takes to subside on rest—angina will usually resolve within seconds or at most a few minutes. If the patient takes glyceryl trinitrate (GTN) tablets, enquire how quickly they seem to work. (Beware—some patients may have a false label of angina, and just because they are taking GTN tablets does not mean that the pain they are describing to you must be angina—a healthy degree of scepticism is useful!) A myocardial infarction usually causes pain lasting for longer than 30 minutes. It would be rash to ascribe such pain to stable angina without other good evidence.

Associated features

Enquire specifically about any associated nausea, vomiting, sweating, shortness of breath, blackout or collapse during the pain. If the patient describes palpitations, it is crucial to know whether they preceded the onset of pain, as occasionally a tachyarrhythmia may cause angina. Establish what the patient means by the term palpitation. Make an attempt to distinguish between angina and myocardial infarction (Fig. 3.3).

Characteristics of angina and myocardial infarction		
Feature	**Angina**	**Myocardial infarction**
site	retrosternal, throat, left arm	retrosternal, throat, left arm
radiation	typically to the throat or left arm.	typically to the throat or left arm
nature	'tight', 'gripping', 'a dull ache'	similar, but usually recognized as more severe
duration	short, usually a few minutes	usually greater than 30 minutes and only terminated by opiate analgesia
precipitation	exertion, stress, cold, emotion	usually none, but may have similar precipitants
relief	rest, GTN (rapid)	often none (opiates)
associated features	usually none	sweating, lightheadedness, palpitations, nausea, vomiting, sense of foreboding

Fig. 3.3 Characteristics of angina and myocardial infarction. (GTN, glyceryl trinitrate.)

Past medical history

Enquire specifically about the major risk factors for ischaemic heart disease:

- Previous episodes of angina or myocardial infarction. Record dates, events, and how the diagnosis was established (e.g. exercise test, hospital admission, angiography).
- Cigarette smoking. 'Pack years' is a useful concept (see Chapter 2). Current smokers have a significantly increased risk compared with ex-smokers.
- Hypertension.
- Diabetes mellitus.
- Hypercholesterolaemia.
- Positive family history of ischaemic heart disease.
- Other vascular disease (e.g. stroke, peripheral vascular disease).

Consider factors other than coronary artery disease that can cause angina (e.g. anaemia, arrhythmia, previous valvular pathology, rheumatic fever).

The major risk factors interact and the probability of ischaemic heart disease is greatly increased if more than one is present.

Drug history

A full list of medication is essential and it is important to note the following:

- Have there been any recent changes?
- The effect of antianginal drugs on symptoms as well as side effects. In particular, does the pain resolve rapidly with sublingual GTN?
- Has compliance been good?
- Is the patient taking aspirin? Check that there are no contraindications (e.g. active ulceration, asthma provoked by aspirin).
- Consider the role of other drugs that might aggravate angina (e.g. theophylline, tricyclic antidepressants, inappropriate dose of thyroxine).

Social history

Enquire whether there have been any recent changes in lifestyle (e.g. financial difficulties, stress at home or work). These outside influences may be the precipitant for angina or a reason for developing a non-cardiac chest pain.

Establish what the baseline exercise tolerance is. Will the patient be able to tolerate an exercise test? Ask how the chest pain has interfered with normal lifestyle.

Review of symptoms

A brief review of symptoms is important for various reasons, including:

- To exclude the gastrointestinal tract as the source of the symptoms (e.g. reflux oesophagitis).
- Associated neurological symptoms may be provoked by decreased perfusion.
- To assess potential risks when considering invasive investigations or treatment (e.g. angiography or thrombolysis).
- To assess whether the patient has the mobility to tolerate an exercise electrocardiogram (ECG).
- To assess whether activity is limited by cardiac status or other factors such as poor mobility, obesity, chronic lung disease.

PALPITATIONS

Presenting complaint

Palpitation is an awareness of the heart beating. Different people mean different things when they say they have experienced palpitations.

Detailed history

It is essential to explore the event in great detail so that the underlying rhythm disturbance and functional consequences can be appreciated.

Nature of the palpitation

It is often possible to make a reasonable estimate of the underlying rhythm from the patient's description (Fig. 3.4), for example in response to questions such as "Can you describe what you experienced?", "Can you tap out the heart beat on the table?"

The rate of the heart during the palpitation often provides a clue to the primary electrical disturbance (Fig. 3.5).

Duration and frequency of episodes

The functional impact on the patient may be revealed as well as the likelihood of being able to 'capture' the event on a 24-hour tape or event recorder.

Associated symptoms

Patients may have symptoms of cardiac decompensation, for example:

- Light-headedness, syncope (due to poor cerebral perfusion and hypotension).
- Chest pain (angina).
- Sweating.

The presence of these symptoms should alert the physician and prompt more detailed investigation.

Characteristics of common arrhythmias causing palpitations	
Rhythm	**Typical features**
ectopic beats	"I felt as though my heart missed a beat"; "a heavy thud"; usually due to awareness of post-extrasystolic beat
atrial fibrillation	'fast, irregular beating'; may be associated with dyspnoea or chest pain, especially if fast rate
supraventricular tachycardia	rapid palpitation, often abrupt onset; may be associated with polyuria; may have rapid termination; patient may have learnt to perform vagal manoeuvres to terminate episode
ventricular tachycardia	often associated with shock, collapse, dyspnoea or progression to cardiac arrest; can be hard to distinguish from supraventricular arrhythmias as features overlap, and may even be asymptomatic; conversely, supraventricular tachycardia can cause shock, especially if rapid

Fig. 3.4 Characteristics of common arrhythmias causing palpitations.

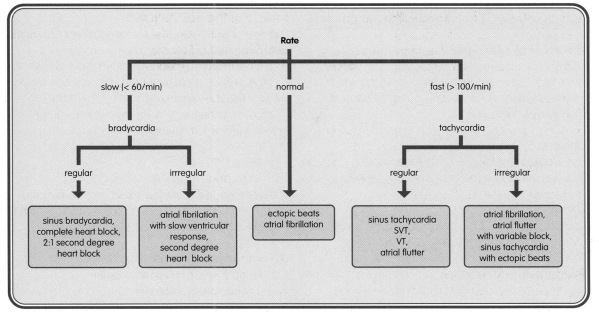

Fig. 3.5 Differential diagnosis of palpitations from the history. (SVT, supraventricular tachycardia; VT, ventricular tachycardia.)

Events immediately preceding palpitation

It is physiological to experience some palpitations after exertion or emotional stress provided they are self-terminating. This may be evident from the response to "What were you doing immediately before the palpitations started?"

If there was chest pain, find out whether the pain preceded the palpitation or coincided with its onset.

Medical history

Review the possible underlying diseases that cause palpitations, including:
- Risk factors for ischaemic heart disease (see p. 21 on chest pain).
- Thyroid disease (especially atrial fibrillation).
- Rheumatic fever.

Drug history

This is very important. Particular attention should be paid to drugs with proarrhythmic effects such as tricyclic antidepressants, digoxin (and other antiarrhythmic agents), and theophylline. Review the response of the palpitations to therapy.

Social history

Particular attention should be paid to consumption of alcohol and caffeine-containing drinks. Use of illicit drugs (e.g. amphetamines) may precipitate arrhythmias.

Summary of aims

The aims of the history for palpitations are as follows:
- The principal aim is to formulate an impression of the underlying electrical disturbance causing the palpitations.
- To distinguish physiological and benign disturbances from potentially serious disorders warranting further investigation and treatment.
- To narrow down the differential diagnosis of the arrhythmia. This is usually possible, but ultimately a diagnosis can only be made by an ECG recording at the time of symptoms.
- To assess whether the episodes are long enough and frequent enough and the patient is capable of using an event recorder or whether a 24-hour ECG is more appropriate if further investigation is needed.

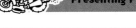

HEART FAILURE

Presenting complaint

Acute
Acute heart failure presents with severe shortness of breath, collapse, severe distress, and production of copious pink, frothy sputum.

Chronic
This presents with fatigue, shortness of breath, limitation of exercise tolerance, and ankle swelling.

Detailed history
The features of heart failure are usually distinctive enough to be recognized from the history alone, but airway obstructions can sometimes be confused with heart failure. The detailed history will clarify the presence of heart failure and establish its severity and possible aetiology.

Chronicity of symptoms
Has the patient had a recent sudden decline suggestive of an ischaemic event? To find out, ask the patient: "When did you last feel perfectly well?" Chart the pattern of deterioration of the symptoms.

Severity of symptoms
Attempt to be quantitative so that a reproducible assessment can be made. Focus on tolerance to exercise and the limiting factor for exercise.

Exercise tolerance
It is often difficult to be precise, but patients may be able to give quantitative answers to questions such as:
- "How many flights of stairs can you climb?"
- "How far can you walk on the flat and uphill?"
- "Do you need help for any activities at home?" Try to ascertain which factor limits exercise capacity (e.g. fatigue, coexisting lung disease, claudication). The severity of the heart failure may be graded according to the New York Heart Association (NYHA) classification (Fig. 3.6).

Limiting factor
Try to establish the limiting symptom for exercise (e.g. dyspnoea, fatigue, chest pain).

Evidence of left heart failure
Enquire about features of pulmonary oedema, for example:
- Paroxysmal nocturnal dyspnoea. This is a feature of acute pulmonary oedema. Ask: "Do you ever wake up in the night fighting for breath?" Patients often describe having to sit upright on the edge of the bed and/or throwing open the windows.
- Orthopnoea. Ask: "How many pillows do you need to sleep with?"

Evidence of right heart failure
Enquire about symptoms related to fluid overload which may result in:
- Ascites.
- Peripheral oedema (in severe cases male patients may have scrotal oedema).
- Right upper quadrant discomfort (due to hepatic congestion).
- Nausea and poor appetite (due to bowel oedema).

Past medical history
The most relevant features include:
- Risk factors for ischaemic heart disease—see Chest pain (cardiac), p. 21.
- Previous cardiac investigations (e.g. echocardiography, angiography, exercise test).
- Other causes of left heart failure (e.g. rheumatic

NHYA grading of severity of heart failure	
Grade	Severity of symptoms
I	unlimited exercise tolerance
II	symptomatic on extra exertion (e.g. stairs)
III	symptomatic on mild exertion (e.g. walking)
IV	symptomatic on minimal exertion or rest (e.g. washing)

Fig. 3.6 The New York Heart Association (NYHA) grading of severity of heart failure provides a simple, but reproducible assessment with interobserver agreement.

fever, valvular disease, cardiomyopathy), high output states (e.g. thyroid disease, Paget's disease, arteriovenous shunt, anaemia).
- Other causes of right heart disease (e.g. chronic lung disease, pulmonary embolus).

Drug history

A full list of medication is needed, but focus on:
- Current therapy for heart failure, for example angiotensin-converting enzyme (ACE) inhibitors (cough may be a side effect or due to mild pulmonary oedema), diuretics (assess compliance and find out whether there has been a recent change in dose).
- Negatively inotropic drugs (e.g. β-blockers, verapamil, class I antiarrhythmic agents).
- Drugs that can induce cardiomyopathy (e.g. doxorubicin).

Social history

This section is very important. Assess daily activities, social support, mobility, etc. Review the patient's diet. Consider salt intake in oedematous states. Does the patient have sufficient mobility to cope with an increased diuresis and avoid incontinence?

DEEP VEIN THROMBOSIS OR PULMONARY EMBOLISM

Presenting complaint

Deep vein thrombosis (DVT) often presents non-specifically, but the most common features include:
- Calf pain.
- Leg swelling.
- Red tender leg.

Pulmonary embolus (PE) may be very difficult to diagnose. The most common presentations are:
- Pleuritic chest pain.
- Shortness of breath.
- Haemoptysis.
- Collapse.

Detailed history

If a PE is suspected, always ask specifically about symptoms suggestive of a DVT. In the presence of calf pain investigate its features systematically (see Chapter 2). In particular, note any preceding symptoms, the speed of onset, any associated symptoms, and whether the pain is unilateral or bilateral. Fig. 3.7 highlights some of the more discriminatory features in the history.

Differential diagnosis of leg swelling or inflammation other than venous thrombosis	
Condition	**Features**
infection (cellulitis)	subacute onset; fever; lymphangitis may be present; ask about portal of entry for infecting organism
ruptured Baker's cyst	preceding arthritis or swelling of knee; acute onset
torn calf muscle	acute onset, often during exercise
Milroy's syndrome (familial lymphatic incompetence)	chronic condition; usually not painful; positive family history
congestive cardiac failure	dyspnoea, fatigue, orthopnoea; risk factors for ischaemic heart disease; usually bilateral leg swelling
lymphatic obstruction	chronic; may be unilateral or bilateral
nephrotic syndrome	subacute or chronic leg swelling; bilateral; usually no features of inflammation

Fig. 3.7 Differential diagnosis of leg swelling or inflammation other than venous thrombosis.

Thromboembolism is treatable and potentially fatal. It is under-recognized. A high index of suspicion is crucial.

Almost 50% of DVTs do not produce local symptoms, so PE may be the presenting feature. Presentation may be non-specific, and the differential diagnosis is wide.

Enquire about risk factors for DVT (an asterisk denotes the more important ones), which include:

- Recent surgery (especially of pelvis or hip)*.
- Pregnancy or puerperium*.
- Prolonged immobility (e.g. long-haul air travel)*.
- Contraceptive pill*.
- Malignancy.
- Family history for antithrombin III deficiency; protein C deficiency (inactivates factors Va and VIIIa); protein S deficiency (regulates activity of protein C); factor V Leiden mutation (probably the most common inherited cause of familial thrombosis).
- Stroke, cardiac failure, nephrotic syndrome, systemic lupus erythematosus.
- Dehydration.

In the presence of pleuritic chest pain of undetermined aetiology, have a low threshold for performing arterial blood gases and obtaining a chest radiograph and an ECG.

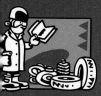

4. Presenting Problems: Respiratory System

ASTHMA

Presenting complaint

The most common presentations include episodic wheeze, shortness of breath or a (nocturnal) cough.

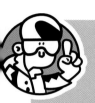

An acute asthma attack is often frightening for both the patient and the attending physician. The patient is often too dyspnoeic to provide much history. The priority is to make a rapid assessment and institute effective therapy. A more detailed history can be obtained once the patient is stable.

Detailed history

If the patient presents with an acute attack, investigate this attack in detail. Obtain a systematic, chronological account of the recent deterioration, focusing on:

- Symptoms (e.g. wheeze, cough, dyspnoea).
- Time course (hours or days).
- Severity—try to quantify in simple terms (e.g. unable to perform vigorous exercise, difficulty climbing stairs, unable to speak a complete sentence, being kept awake at night).
- Onset and precipitating events (e.g. exercise, emotional stress, viral illness, house dust, pets).
- Intervention during present attack, and response (e.g. nebulized bronchodilators, glucocorticosteroids).
- Reason for seeking medical attention at this stage.

Often asthma control has deteriorated chronically and insidiously. Ask either:
- "Is there anything that you could do six months ago that you couldn't manage before this attack?"
- "Have you reduced your exercise over the past few months?"

Past medical history
Baseline asthma control

It is helpful to gain an awareness of the background control—in addition to allowing an assessment of disease severity, it may reveal information about the patient's understanding of the disease. Ask about:

- Usual exercise tolerance. Try to quantify as described above. (Young patients should have unlimited exercise capacity. Older patients often have coexisting morbidity.)
- Frequency of attacks.
- Best recorded peak expiratory flow rate (PEFR). All asthma patients should have their own peak flow meter and know their baseline PEFR.
- Usual precipitating factors (e.g. pollen, stress, exercise, dust, pollution).
- Usual medication (see below).
- Usual response to therapy during exacerbations. For example, ask: "Is this the worst attack you've ever had?", "Would you normally expect your asthma attacks to get better after a nebulizer?"
- Previous hospital admissions. For example, ask: "Have you ever been admitted to hospital with asthma?", "Have you ever needed to be put on an artificial ventilator?"
- Symptoms suggestive of poor baseline control. This is very important and under-recognized. (e.g. 'morning dips', poor sleep, nocturnal cough, time off work or school). An example of a peak flow chart from a child with poor control is illustrated in Fig. 4.1.

Other atopic conditions

Ask about other atopic conditions such as eczema, hay fever, urticaria.

Coexisting respiratory disease

Coexisting respiratory disease is particularly important in patients who present later in life as it may be hard to distinguish asthma from chronic obstructive pulmonary disease (COPD) from the history.

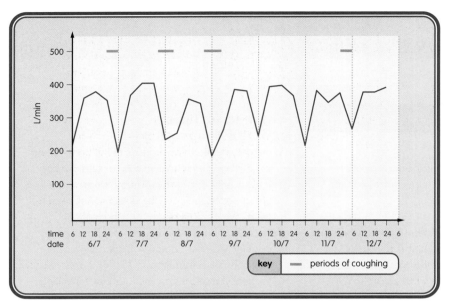

Fig. 4.1 An example of a peak flow recording from an adolescent with poor asthma control. Note the presence of cough at night and 'morning dips'.

Drug history

Obtain a full list of medication. Ask specifically about:
- Bronchodilators.
- Theophylline or aminophylline (phosphodiesterase inhibitors). Have the drug levels ever been measured?
- Glucocorticosteroids.

Ask patients to demonstrate their inhaler technique.

Find out whether lung function tests have been performed to assess airway reversibility, and responses to different agents, especially for older patients for whom it may be difficult to define the relative components of asthma and COPD to the overall morbidity.

Consider medication that may aggravate the symptoms (e.g. β-blockers, aspirin).

Social history

Review how the asthma is interfering with lifestyle for both older and young patients (e.g. school activities, absenteeism from work, limitation in sports, difficulty walking to the shops).

Always specifically enquire about smoking. During an exacerbation, it is timely to offer sensitive advice about smoking! Ask whether anyone in the patient's household is a smoker.

No one with asthma should smoke!

Review of systems enquiry

Focus on other diseases that may limit exercise tolerance, especially cardiovascular and respiratory pathology.

Remember that asthma is a potentially fatal disease. The morbidity and mortality are high, and can be overcome by better supervision, objective assessment, better patient understanding and participation in his or her management, and appropriate use of glucocorticosteroids.

CHRONIC OBSTRUCTIVE PULMONARY DISEASE (COPD)

Detailed history

Obtain a detailed history of chest symptoms. Patients usually present with an acute deterioration of dyspnoea in association with a productive cough. Outline a detailed history of the present attack following the usual systematic approach to explore:

- Time course.
- Treatment given and effects.
- Functional impact on lifestyle.

Obtain a thorough history of baseline function trying to be as objective as possible, for example ask:

- "Can you walk 100 yards on the flat?"
- "Can you climb one flight of stairs easily?"
- "Do you get short of breath dressing?"
- "Did you manage to walk to the outpatients department without stopping?"

It is typical for a patient with COPD to have a pattern of chronically deteriorating exercise tolerance punctuated with acute declines during an infective exacerbation (Fig. 4.2). These may be seasonal, with an increased frequency in the winter months.

Sputum production and cough are characteristic. Try to quantify the usual amount and its characteristics (e.g. teaspoonful, eggcupful).

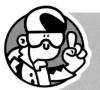

Chronic bronchitis is defined on the basis of a cough that produces sputum on the majority of days in three consecutive months for at least two years. Emphysema is a pathological diagnosis of dilatation and destruction of the lungs distal to the terminal bronchioles. In practice, these conditions coexist.

Consider the possibility of cor pulmonale in a patient with severe disease who describes ankle swelling.

Ascertain aggravating factors (e.g. cold weather, pollution, exertion).

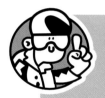

Many patients with COPD have a reversible component to their disease. This is under-recognized, but can be uncovered by a formal trial of glucocorticosteroids.

Find out whether a satisfactory attempt has been made to establish the diagnosis, for example:

- Have lung function tests been performed to assess airway reversibility?
- Have arterial blood gases been assessed?

A useful time to check arterial blood gases is when the patient is stable (e.g. on discharge from a hospital admission or in an outpatient clinic).

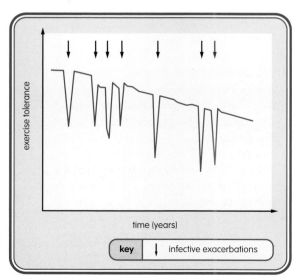

| key | ↓ infective exacerbations |

Fig. 4.2 Exercise tolerance in a patient with COPD.

Past medical history

These patients often have multiple medical problems, which should be recorded, but specifically ask about:

- Previous admissions to hospital with acute exacerbations of COPD. Record the frequency, especially within the last year.
- Other smoking-related diseases (e.g. ischaemic heart disease, peripheral vascular disease, strokes, hypertension).
- Other causes of lung disease (e.g. occupational exposure to dusts, bronchiectasis due to, for example, previous tuberculosis, childhood whooping cough).
- Asthma. There may be a reversible component to the disease.

Drug history

Review medication prescribed for COPD, for example:

- Bronchodilators (inhalers and nebulizers).
- Home oxygen. Who initiated therapy and on what evidence? How many hours a day is it being used?
- Theophylline. Have blood levels been measured recently?
- Glucocorticosteroids. Does the patient have a steroid card?

Review inhaler technique.

Social history

This is particularly important for these patients as they often have a significantly limited exercise tolerance and rely heavily upon support from family and friends. Consider all aspects of daily living.

A detailed occupational history may be important if there is any doubt about the patient's ability to continue working or the aetiology of the lung disease, for example:

- Exposure to inorganic dusts (coalminer's lung, silicosis, asbestosis).
- Occupational asthma (isocyanates, colophony fumes).
- Extrinsic allergic bronchiolar alveolitis (farmworkers, 'bird fanciers').

Obtain a detailed smoking history as this is undoubtedly a smoking-related disease in the vast majority of patients. Remember that it is dangerous to smoke if you are using home oxygen!

Review of systems enquiry

Many patients with COPD have multiple pathologies related to their smoking, so a thorough trawl of their symptoms may raise suspicions of previously unrecognized conditions (e.g. ischaemic heart disease, malignancy, renal disease, peripheral vascular disease).

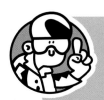

A meticulous and realistic assessment of baseline function is essential—without this, it is impossible to make difficult decisions about appropriate treatment and to set realistic goals of therapy.

CHEST INFECTION

Detailed history

Perform a detailed enquiry about presenting symptoms, adopting a methodical approach. Ask specifically about symptoms referable to the respiratory tract, as follows:

- Cough—duration, whether productive or dry.
- Sputum production—quantity, colour, recent changes if the patient has a productive cough.
- Dyspnoea—obtain a quantitative account of exercise tolerance at baseline and during the current illness.
- Wheeze.
- Pleuritic chest pain—a common feature of pneumonia, but be aware of the possibility of a pulmonary embolus.
- Fever.

Clues to the underlying cause of pneumonia	
Organism	**Features from history**
Streptococcus pneumoniae*	most frequent identifiable infecting organism in community-acquired pneumonia; associated with herpes labialis; commonly prominent fever and pleuritic pain; often abrupt onset in previously fit individual
Mycoplasma pneumoniae*	occurs in epidemics with a 3–4-year periodicity; usually occurs in previously fit people; often young adults; may be preceded by a prodromal illness with headache and malaise; may be prominent extrapulmonary features (e.g. nausea, vomiting, myalgia, rash)
Haemophilus influenzae*	most common bacterial pneumonia following influenza; associated with underlying lung disease (especially COPD)
Legionella pneumophila	associated with institutional outbreaks (e.g. hospitals, hotels); may be associated with mental confusion or gastrointestinal symptoms; typically causes a dry cough
Coxiella burnetii	contact with farm animals
Chlamydia psittaci	contact with infected birds ("Do you have a sick parrot?")
Staphylococcus aureus	associated with preceding influenza, intravenous drug abusers; patient is often very ill
Gram-negative organisms	hospitalized patients; may be community-acquired in elderly or diabetics; Branhamella catarrhalis is associated with exacerbations of COPD
Pneumocystis carinii, cytomegalovirus, Nocardia asteroides, Mycobacterium avium intracellulare	acquired immunodeficiency syndrome (AIDS); transplant recipients; chemotherapy

Fig. 4.3 Clues to the underlying cause of pneumonia. * denotes the more common organisms.

Ask about associated symptoms that may have immediately preceded or coincided with the illness (especially gastrointestinal). These may give additional clues to the infecting organism causing pneumonia. Fig. 4.3 illustrates how a detailed history may help to identify the microbiological cause of a pneumonic illness.

Drug history
Ask specifically about antibiotics used to treat this episode, and the duration of use, as the response to therapy may give a clue to the infecting agent as well as the likelihood of obtaining a positive blood culture, for example:
- Resistance of Mycoplasma to penicillin.
- Resistance of Mycobacterium tuberculosis or Pneumocystis to repeated courses of antibiotics.

Ask patients whether they are taking immunosuppressive medication (e.g. those taking glucocorticosteroids, transplant recipients) (Fig. 4.4).

Social history

Relevant clues may be provided by a travel history and details of hobbies (e.g. involving pets), occupation, and risk factors (e.g. for HIV infection). Smokers are more likely to decompensate earlier in the course of the illness. Clearly, it is important to assess the functional impact of the disease on patients and their families so that appropriate therapeutic and management decisions can be made.

 If symptoms are prolonged, recurrent, or associated with weight loss, consider the possibility of an underlying malignancy, especially in a smoker.

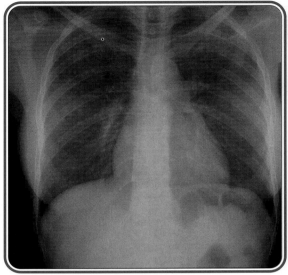

Fig. 4.4 Radiograph of a patient with *Pneumocystis* pneumonia. Note the reticulonodular shadowing with characteristic sparing of the peripheries. *Pneumocystis* pneumonia occurs in the presence of immunosuppression.

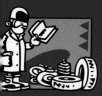

5. Presenting Problems: Abdominal

ACUTE ABDOMINAL PAIN

Detailed history

A very careful history needs to be elicited as it will form the foundation for a working hypothesis and differential diagnosis, and hence subsequent investigation.

On the basis of the history, abdominal pain can be divided into three types:

- Visceral.
- Somatic.
- Referred.

Visceral (deep) pain

This is dull, poorly localized pain referred to the midline. The site of pain is derived from its embryological origin (foregut, midgut, hindgut) (Fig. 5.1).

Somatic (peritoneal) pain

This is sharp, severe, and more precisely localized pain. It occurs when the disease process involves the surrounding peritoneum and mesentery.

Referred pain

This is the perception of sensory stimuli at a distance from its source (e.g. acute cholecystitis causing diaphragmatic irritation with the patient feeling pain over the right shoulder tip). The characteristics of the pain should be reviewed in a systematic manner as for other forms of pain (e.g. see 'Chest pain', p.19). There are several key areas that should always be investigated.

Site of the pain

Define the initial location of the pain and whether it has subsequently moved (e.g. as is common in acute appendicitis). This is of great importance as certain disease processes tend to cause pain localized to a defined region of the abdomen (Fig. 5.2).

Time and mode of onset

Sudden-onset pain suggests a vascular event (e.g. rupture of an abdominal aortic aneurysm), or perforation of a viscus: "One moment I was feeling fine, the next I had excruciating pain!"

Frequency and duration

Colicky pain occurs when there is a pathological process in a smooth muscular tube (e.g. small and large bowel, ureter, fallopian tube). Ask whether the patient has had previous similar episodes.

Character

The pain may change character, indicating progression of the pathology (e.g. transition of colicky pain to constant pain suggests transition of visceral to peritoneal involvement in acute appendicitis).

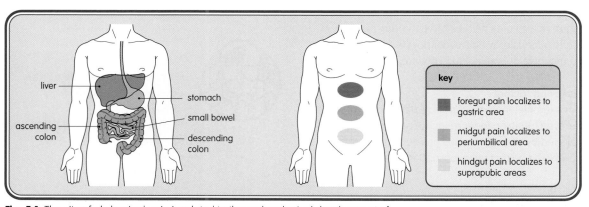

Fig. 5.1 The site of abdominal pain is related to the embryological development of the foregut, midgut, and hindgut.

key

█ foregut pain localizes to gastric area

█ midgut pain localizes to periumbilical area

░ hindgut pain localizes to suprapubic areas

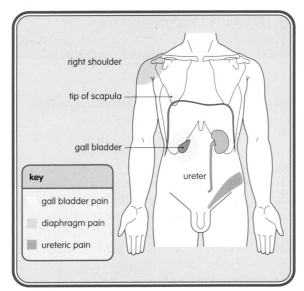

Fig. 5.2 Typical sites of radiation for pain originating in the gall bladder, diaphragm, and ureter.

Severity

Is the pain getting worse, better, or staying at the same intensity? "If 0 equals no pain, and 10 is the worst pain you have ever experienced, what value would you give this pain?"

Radiation

For example loin pain radiates to the groin in renal or ureteric colic.

Aggravating factors

It is often apparent from first seeing patients what type of pain they have (e.g. patients with peritonitis lie still, patients with ureteric colic are often very restless). Certain foods may aggravate pain (e.g. fatty foods aggravates abdominal pain due to gallstones).

Relieving factors

For example, the pain of pancreatitis is characteristically relieved by sitting forward; duodenal ulcer pain may be relieved by eating; antacids or sleeping upright may relieve the pain of reflux oesophagitis.

Cause

Ask the patient what he or she thinks is the cause of the pain.

Other symptoms

Review other symptoms referable to the abdominal system:

- When did the patient last defecate and when was flatus last passed? This is particularly relevant if partial or complete obstruction is suspected.
- Change in bowel habit. This is likely to reflect a large bowel pathology (e.g. carcinoma, inflammatory bowel disease—see p. 44).
- Vomiting. Establish the nature of the vomitus (i.e. blood, bile, 'coffee grounds', faeculent).
- "Do you still feel hungry?" This is useful for discriminating non-serious pathology as the majority of patients with serious intra-abdominal disease have anorexia.
- Abdominal distension.
- Appetite and weight loss. Chronic weight loss is suggestive of an underlying malignancy.
- Dysphagia. Ask the patient to point to where the food appears to stick. Establish whether the dysphagia is for food or both food and drink. Enquire whether there is associated pain on swallowing.
- Regurgitation, flatulence, heartburn, dyspepsia. Ask about these symptoms if there is a suspected peptic ulcer, gastro-oesophageal reflux or gallstone disease.
- Sore throat or influenza. Young children may have associated abdominal pain, which can be hard to distinguish from acute appendicitis.
- Urinary symptoms. Frequency and dysuria may suggest a urinary tract infection. Nocturia, urgency, and hesitancy are consistent with prostatic enlargement.
- History of trauma. Have a high index of suspicion for a splenic or hepatic tear.

Remember the six Fs as the causes of abdominal distension:
- **Fat.**
- **Fluid.**
- **Faeces.**
- **Foetus.**
- **Fibroids.**
- **Flatus.**

Obtain a gynaecological history from women as gynaecological pathology often presents as acute abdominal pain. Ask about:

- Menstrual cycle. Time of last period, duration of cycle, mid-cycle pain (mittelschmerz) or dysmenorrhoea (endometriosis).
- Vaginal discharge. This may suggest pelvic inflammatory disease.
- Dyspareunia (pain during sexual intercourse). Causes include pelvic inflammatory disease, endometriosis.
- Pregnancies.

Consider the possibility of pregnancy in all women of childbearing age.

It is particularly important to include a cardiovascular and respiratory history as several medical conditions can cause acute abdominal pain (Fig. 5.3).

Past medical history

Obtain a detailed history, paying particular attention to:

- Previous operations—adhesions, recurrent pathology, etc.
- Recent myocardial infarction or cardiac arrhythmias—mesenteric embolus, especially in association with atrial fibrillation.
- Psychiatric history—pseudo-obstruction, sigmoid volvulus, porphyria, Munchausen syndrome.
- Hypothyroidism—constipation.

Drug history

Obtain a full list of medication. Pay attention to non-steroidal anti-inflammatory drugs (NSAIDs) and glucocorticosteroids. Also consider drugs that may provoke constipation (e.g. opiates, tricyclic antidepressants, antimuscarinic agents, antiparkinsonism therapy).

Family history

There may be a positive family history of inflammatory bowel disease or bowel carcinoma.

Medical conditions that can mimic a 'surgical abdomen'	
Medical condition presenting as abdominal pain	**Features**
myocardial infarction (MI)*	especially inferior MI; may have paradoxical bradycardia; risk factors for ischaemic heart disease
angina*	usually epigastric
chest infection*	especially lower lobe pneumonia; previous respiratory symptoms; pleurisy
diabetic ketoacidosis*	especially young patient; decreased level of consciousness; preceding polyuria, polydipsia, weight loss; positive family history
acute pyelonephritis*	dysuria, haematuria, frequency; loin pain versus central abdominal pain; history of renal stones
hypercalcaemia	often elderly; 'bones, stones, moans and groans'
sickle cell crisis	ethnic origin; usually known history
lead poisoning	rare
porphyria	rare; occasionally strong alcohol history (porphyria cutanea tarda)

Fig. 5.3 Medical conditions that can mimic a 'surgical abdomen'. The history may distinguish medical conditions masquerading as surgical problems.
* indicates the more common conditions.

Social history

Alcohol history is extremely important (e.g. for peptic ulcer, pancreatitis). For diarrhoeal illnesses consider foreign travel (e.g. amoebiasis, typhoid, giardiasis) or food poisoning (ask "Are any of your friends or family also affected?").

If the patient may need an operation, do not forget to ask when he or she last had food or drink.

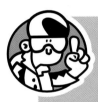

In the majority of cases it is kinder to give analgesia at the earliest opportunity. It rarely makes interpretation of physical signs difficult, and patients give better histories if they are less distracted.

- Allergy to gluten products.
- Symptoms of thyrotoxicosis (e.g. heat intolerance, agitation, palpitations); thyrotoxicosis occasionally presents with diarrhoea.

Past medical history

Obtain a detailed history, paying particular attention to:
- Previous operations (e.g. short bowel syndrome, gastrectomy and post-vagotomy dumping).
- Inflammatory bowel disease.

Drug history

This is particularly important as drugs commonly contribute to a diarrhoeal state. Common culprits include antibiotics, laxative abuse (may be surreptitious), and magnesium-containing antacids.

Family history

Enquire about inflammatory bowel disease, carcinoma of the bowel, coeliac disease.

Social history

An infective aetiology is suggested if friends or relatives have a similar illness. If the patient is dehydrated, frail,

ACUTE DIARRHOEAL ILLNESS

Detailed history

Diarrhoea is a symptom and not a disease. Therefore it is important to establish the underlying cause. Ask about the nature of the stools, frequency, and events surrounding the episode. Important features to ask about include:
- Recent ingestion of undercooked meat, shellfish, unpasteurized milk, stream water (i.e. food poisoning).
- Associated abdominal pain and vomiting. Is the patient likely to need intravenous fluids?
- Is the pain relieved by defecation?
- Is there blood, pus, or mucus in the stool?
- Are the stools pale and frothy (i.e. steatorrhoea).
- Duration of symptoms (e.g. hours, weeks, days—different illnesses may present acutely or subacutely).
- Weight loss or anorexia.
- Recent return from a foreign country (e.g. amoebiasis, giardiasis).

Causes of diarrhoea
infective viral, *Salmonella,* *Shigella,* *Campylobacter,* enterotoxic *Escherichia coli,* *Entamoeba histolytica* (if appropriate travel history), *Clostridium difficile* (if recent use of broad-spectrum antibiotics)
inflammatory bowel disease
colorectal carcinoma
coeliac disease
drugs
anxiety states
miscellaneous thyrotoxicosis, Zollinger–Ellison syndrome (very rare), carcinoid syndrome (rare)

Fig. 5.4 Causes of diarrhoea.

or responsible for child care consider whether hospital admission is indicated.

The more common causes of diarrhoea are listed in Fig. 5.4.

JAUNDICE

Presenting complaint

Jaundice presents with yellow discolouration, which is often not noticed by the patient.

Detailed history

The history of a jaundiced patient is very challenging as the pathophysiology is so varied. It is helpful to review the pathophysiology of jaundice (Figs 5.5 and 5.6). Focus on the major features.

Onset

Who noticed the jaundice? (e.g. patient, family, abnormal blood test). Establish the time course (e.g. acute onset in fulminant hepatitis A, insidious progression in biliary stricture).

Associated symptoms

It is often possible to narrow down the differential diagnosis of jaundice by a detailed history. Many causes of jaundice have typical features. The usual classification is prehepatic, hepatocellular and posthepatic. Often the features of hepatocellular and obstructive jaundice overlap.

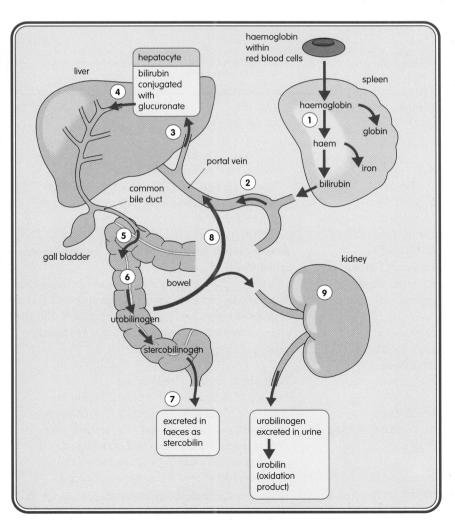

Fig. 5.5 The production, circulation, and clearance of bilirubin (see Fig. 5.6).

	Production and clearance of bilirubin	
Stage	**Description**	**Example of pathology**
1	haemoglobin within the red cells broken down within the spleen producing non-water-soluble unconjugated bilirubin.	excessive breakdown (e.g. haemolytic anaemia)
2	unconjugated bilirubin transported in the blood to the liver	
3	uptake of bilirubin by the hepatocytes and transfer to the smooth endoplasmic reticulum	drug toxicity; Gilbert's syndrome; Rotor's syndrome
4	conjugation with glucuronate	Crigler–Najjar syndrome
5	excretion of conjugated bilirubin in the bile into the small bowel	biliary obstruction (defect may occur at level of hepatocyte, bile canaliculi, or bile duct)
6	breakdown within bowel to stercobilinogen (urobilinogen)	
7	oxidation of stercobilinogen to stercobilin (causes brown colouration of faeces) and excretion	white stool in cholestatic jaundice
8	absorption of urobilinogen; most goes through enterohepatic recirculation	
9	small amount of urobilinogen (water soluble) reaches systemic circulation and excreted via the kidney	large amounts of urinary urobilinogen detectable if severe haemolysis or liver damage saturates the liver's capacity for enterohepatic recirculation

Fig. 5.6 Production and clearance of bilirubin. Stage refers to Fig. 5.5.

Prehepatic jaundice (haemolytic)

Jaundice is usually a minor component of the illness. The illness is often dominated by symptoms of anaemia, for example fatigue, dyspnoea, angina, and palpitations (in older patients). It may be associated with gallstones (pigment stones). On specific questioning patients report normal-coloured stool and urine. Patients may be transfusion dependent. Consider the possible causes (i.e. abnormal red cells or immune-mediated haemolysis).

Examples of abnormal red cells occur in:
- Congenital spherocytosis (Northern Europe).
- Glucose-6-phosphate dehydrogenase (G6PD) deficiency (West Africa, Mediterranean, Middle East, Southeast Asia).
- Sickle-cell anaemia (sub-Saharan Africa).
- Thalassaemia (Mediterranean, Middle East, India, Southeast Asia).

Causes of immune-mediated haemolysis include:
- Drugs (e.g. methyldopa, penicillin).
- Incompatible blood transfusion (acute onset).

- Warm autoantibodies (e.g. systemic lupus erythematosus, lymphoproliferative disorders).
- Cold agglutinins (e.g. infectious mononucleosis, *Mycoplasma*).

Hepatocellular jaundice (inability to excrete bilirubin into the bile)

This is often dominated by symptoms of liver dysfunction (e.g. malaise, anorexia, right upper quadrant discomfort, abdominal distension, loss of libido, confusion). The list of diseases that may be responsible is vast, but the more important causes are illustrated in Fig. 5.7.

Posthepatic jaundice (cholestatic)

The patient may complain of pruritus due to the deposition of bile salts. It is usually, but not always, relentlessly progressive rather than episodic. There is often a history of pale stools and dark urine due to a lack of stercobilinogen in the stool and retention of conjugated bilirubin. It is important to recognize extrahepatic causes of obstructive jaundice as these are often amenable to surgical intervention (Fig. 5.8).

Fig. 5.7 Causes of hepatocellular jaundice. * indicates the more common causes.

Causes of hepatocellular jaundice	
Cause	**Examples**
viral*	hepatitis A* (common, especially in endemic areas. may occur in epidemics; may present acutely); hepatitis B* (common in endemic areas, e.g. Southeast Asia; ask specifically about risk factors for bloodborne infections); hepatitis C* (becoming more common; ask about blood transfusions, shared needles in drug addicts; usually chronic insidious illness)
alcoholic*	common; often presents as acute hepatitic illness
drugs*	common in hospitalized patients (e.g. rifampicin, isoniazid, prolonged course of antibiotics, paracetamol overdose, etc.)
cirrhosis*	of any aetiology (e.g. alcohol, biliary, haemochromatosis, etc.)
malignant infiltration*	primary or secondary (especially bronchus, bowel, breast)
congenital	for example Gilbert's syndrome* (common and mild); Crigler–Najjar syndrome
acute fatty liver of pregnancy	rare
inherited disorders	for example α-1-antitrypsin deficiency, Wilson's disease, etc.

Fig. 5.8 Causes of posthepatic jaundice. * indicates the more common causes.

Causes of post-hepatic jaundice	
Cause	**Features from the history**
gallstones*	common; often intermittent history of biliary colic or rigors; 'fat, female, forty, fertile'
carcinoma of head of pancreas*	weight loss; pain; relentless progression
pancreatitis*	acute onset; patient often very ill
benign stricture of common bile duct	may mimic carcinoma of the pancreas
sclerosing cholangitis	associated ulcerative colitis
cholangiocarcinoma	

Past medical history

Obtain a detailed history, paying particular attention to more recent events, for example:

- Recent surgery—halothane hepatotoxicity.
- Ulcerative colitis—may suggest the presence of sclerosing cholangitis.
- Recent viral illness—Gilbert's syndrome, hepatitis A or B.
- Gallstones—either a cause of jaundice or a consequence of chronic haemolysis.

Drug history

An extremely careful drug history should be taken as drugs may have precipitated the jaundice. In addition certain drugs need to be avoided or used with care in liver disease. For example:

- Drugs causing haemolysis—acting as hapten (e.g. penicillin, sulphonamides), direct autoimmune effect (e.g. methyldopa), precipitating haemolysis in G6PD deficiency (e.g. primaquine, nitrofurantoin).
- Drugs causing hepatocellular damage—for example paracetamol overdose, alcohol, isoniazid.

37

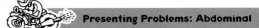
- Drugs causing intrahepatic cholestasis—for example oestrogens, phenothiazines.
- Drugs causing gallstones—for example oral contraceptives, clofibrate.

Social history

Reviewing the patient's lifestyle may provide many clues to the aetiology. A travel history is particularly pertinent (e.g. to an area where hepatitis A is endemic). Risk factors for bloodborne infections (e.g. intravenous drug abuse, homosexual intercourse, unprotected sexual intercourse, multiple blood transfusions) should be considered (e.g. for hepatitis B or C, HIV infection). A detailed alcohol history is essential for acute alcoholic hepatitis and cirrhosis. Cigarette smoking may point to malignant disease. Social contacts with hepatitis A may be apparent if there has been an epidemic.

Finally review the patient's occupation and hobbies (e.g. leptospirosis in sewage workers or farmers, exposure to toxins by workers with organic solvents, hepatitis B in health care workers on dialysis units).

Family history

A family history is particularly relevant for younger patients (e.g. for Gilbert's syndrome, haemoglobinopathies, Wilson's disease).

Review of systems enquiry

The differential diagnosis is broad, so a complete systems enquiry is needed.

The differential diagnosis of jaundice is broad. A detailed history is needed to focus further investigations.

ANAEMIA

Presenting complaint

Examples include lethargy, pallor, or an incidental finding on blood test.

Detailed history

Review symptoms related to anaemia. Ask specifically about:
- Lethargy.

- Exercise tolerance.
- Palpitations.
- Angina and intermittent claudication (older patients).
- Dyspnoea.

Try to establish the duration of symptoms; the causes of acute and chronic anaemia are different. For example, ask: "When did you last feel completely well?" Obtain the results of previous laboratory investigations—they may help in differentiating acute and chronic causes (Fig. 5.9).

Usually the result of the blood film will be available. It is helpful to categorize anaemia according to the mean corpuscular volume (MCV) (Fig. 5.10) as:
- Hypochromic microcytic.
- Normochromic normocytic.
- Macrocytic.

Past medical history

Take an extensive history. Ask specifically about the following conditions, including symptoms relating to:
- Peptic ulceration or indigestion—blood loss causing iron deficiency.
- Malignancy—chronic disease, marrow infiltration, blood loss.
- Renal disease—chronic disease, blood loss, haemolysis, erythropoietin deficiency.
- Connective tissue diseases.
- Thyroid disease—previous treatment with radioiodine.
- Diseases associated with pernicious anaemia—for example Addison's disease, vitiligo, diabetes mellitus, thyroiditis.
- Jaundice—alcohol abuse, chronic liver disease, haemolysis.

Drug history

A particularly detailed drug history is important as drugs can often cause or exacerbate anaemia. Drugs can cause anaemia in many ways, for example:
- Blood loss—aspirin or NSAIDs.
- Haemolysis—immune-mediated (e.g. quinidine, methyldopa), G6PD deficiency (e.g. antimalarials, dapsone, favism).
- Aplasia—cytotoxic chemotherapy, idiopathic (e.g. sulphonamides).
- Megaloblastic anaemia—phenytoin, dihydrofolate reductase inhibitors (trimethoprim, methotrexate).
- Sideroblastic anaemia—isoniazid.

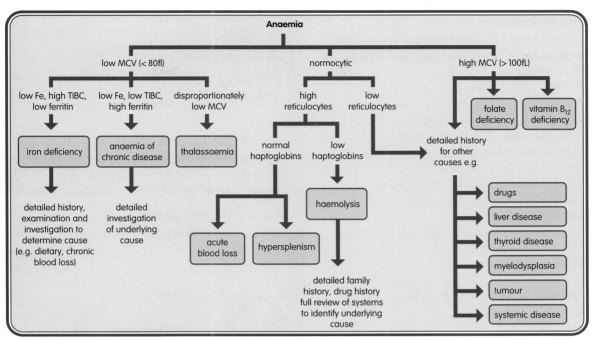

Fig. 5.9 Algorithm for the differential diagnosis of anaemia based on the mean corpuscular volume (MCV). (Fe, iron; TIBC, total iron-binding capacity; fl, fento litre, the unit of MCV))

Causes of anaemia	
Causes	**Features**
hypochromic	
iron deficiency*	overwhelmingly the most common cause of anaemia; usually a chronic insidious pattern (e.g. dietary, chronic blood loss)
thalassaemia trait and disease	disproportionately low MCV; Mediterranean; family history
anaemia of chronic disease*	may have normal MCV
congenital sideroblastic anaemia	rare
normochromic normocytic	
haemolytic anaemia*	often variable red cell indices;
aplastic anaemia	may have variable MCV due to reticulocytosis (e.g. G6PD deficiency, drug-induced, etc.)
anaemia of chronic disease	usually multifactorial causes (e.g. malignancy, chronic renal failure, connective tissue disease, etc.)
macrocytic	
vitamin B_{12} deficiency*	common, megaloblastic (e.g. pernicious anaemia, veganism)
folate deficiency*	common, megaloblastic (e.g. nutritional, malabsorption, pregnancy)
alcohol*	the most common cause of an elevated MCV
hypothyroidism	
liver disease	
reticulocytosis	
myelodysplasia	rare
acquired sideroblastic anaemia	rare

Fig. 5.10 Causes of anaemia. * indicates the more common causes. (G6PD, glucose-6-phosphate-dehydrogenase.)

Family history

Consider the possibility of an inherited haemolytic anaemia (especially in the appropriate ethnic group), for example:

- Sickle-cell anaemia—especially in sub-Saharan Africans and malarial areas.
- Thalassaemia—especially in those from the Mediterranean, Middle East, India, Southeast Asia.
- Hereditary spherocytosis—Northern Europeans.
- G6PD deficiency—in people from West Africa, Mediterranean, Middle East, Southeast Asia.

Social history

Focus on the diet, especially if there is iron, folate, or vitamin B_{12} deficiency. In addition, alcohol can cause anaemia in many ways.

Review of systems enquiry

As the cause of anaemia is often multifactorial, the systems enquiry is often fruitful. In particular, consider causes of chronic blood loss (e.g. dyspepsia, melaena, menorrhagia) and symptoms suggestive of systemic disease (e.g. weight loss, fevers, sweats).

If a particular cause of anaemia is suspected, specific questions relating to that system should be asked in detail.

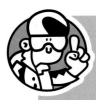

Anaemia is often multifactorial, so a detailed history is essential to elucidate different components. A diagnosis of 'iron deficiency' is inadequate. The underlying cause for the deficiency must be found.

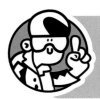

A useful starting point for detailed history taking is the MCV.

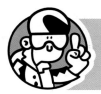

Always ask about the use of aspirin or NSAIDs.

MELAENA AND ACUTE GASTROINTESTINAL BLEEDING

Presenting complaint

Typical presentations include haematemesis, dyspepsia, abdominal pain, and 'tarry black stools'.

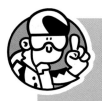

The presence of melaena indicates that the source of blood loss is probably proximal to and including the caecum. Conversely, the presence of discernible blood per rectum does not necessarily imply a distal source of blood loss if the loss is brisk.

Detailed history

The most common causes of acute gastrointestinal (GI) bleeding include the following, those with an asterisk being the most common:

- Gastric ulcer*.
- Duodenal ulcer*.
- Gastric erosions and gastritis*.
- Mallory–Weiss syndrome.
- Oesophageal varices.
- Haemorrhagic peptic oesophagitis.
- Gastric carcinoma (rarely presents with an acute GI bleed).
- Hereditary haemorrhagic telangiectasia (rare).

The patient presenting with GI bleeding is often shocked, and the immediate priority is to perform adequate resuscitation before obtaining a thorough history.

Ask specifically about symptoms suggestive of haemodynamic instability, including:

- Faintness and loss of consciousness.
- Sweating.
- Palpitations.
- Confusion.

Obtain a detailed history, focusing on symptoms referable to the gastrointestinal tract. Ask specifically about abdominal pain, dyspepsia and heartburn, vomiting and nausea, weight loss, and early satiety.

Ask about the duration of symptoms. It is worth enquiring whether the patient has experienced any symptoms suggestive of anaemia (e.g. lethargy, angina, palpitations, unexplained fatigue).

There may be a periodicity and relationship to food or identifiable precipitating events, for example an alcoholic binge, vomiting (e.g. Mallory–Weiss syndrome, pyloric stenosis).

Medical history

Ask about pre-existing GI tract pathologies and investigations (e.g. endoscopy, barium meal). Liver disease or jaundice may suggest gastritis or oesophageal varices in the presence of portal hypertension.

Drug history

Ask specifically about:

- Aspirin and NSAIDs (common causes of gastritis).
- Glucocorticosteroids (may exacerbate pre-existing ulcer).
- Use of antacids, histamine H_2 blockers, proton pump inhibitors.

Family history

Patients with peptic ulceration often have a positive family history.

Social history

Cigarettes are associated with peptic ulceration. Alcohol is strongly associated with liver disease and gastritis. Binge drinkers may have been vomiting and produced Mallory–Weiss tears.

The underlying cause of the bleed is often indicated from the history, but subsequent confirmation by endoscopy is almost invariably indicated.

CHANGE IN BOWEL HABIT

Presenting complaint

Patients may present with either a change in normal stool frequency or a change in the nature of the stool.

Detailed history

The main conditions producing a change in bowel habit are illustrated in Fig. 5.11. Find out what the normal pattern of bowel movements are for the patient. A normal pattern varies from one stool every three days to three stools a day. Enquire specifically about the frequency of stools and do not accept terms such as 'diarrhoea' or 'constipation' without clarification.

Ask about the duration of symptoms. A very short history of a few hours is likely to indicate an infective aetiology, whereas altered bowel habit for many years is more likely to indicate inflammatory bowel disease in a young patient. Ask specifically about weight loss, anorexia, fatigue, and their onset.

Associated abdominal pain may suggest an anatomical site of pathology (e.g. left iliac fossa pain is common with disease of the sigmoid colon).

Enquire about the presence of blood in the stool (Fig. 5.12). The colour and relationship to the stool may reveal its origin as follows:

- Bright red blood on the surface of the stool occurs with rectosigmoid lesions (e.g. polyp, carcinoma) or haemorrhoids.

Causes of change in bowel habit	
Condition	**Features**
colorectal carcinoma	weight loss; chronic history; blood in the stool
inflammatory bowel disease	Crohn's disease; ulcerative colitis; ask about systemic manifestations (e.g. arthropathy, oral ulcers, weight loss, etc.)
diverticular disease	very common; older patients; hard to diagnose from the history and examination alone
colonic polyps	may have mucoid discharge
infective colitis	usually acute, explosive history
irritable bowel syndrome	colicky abdominal pain; bloating; mucus; related to stress; absence of any sinister features in the history; very common

Fig. 5.11 Causes of change in bowel habit.

- Red blood mixed with the stool is a feature of colorectal lesions (e.g. polyp, carcinoma, inflammatory bowel disease, diverticular disease).
- Altered blood or clots almost always implies significant pathology (e.g. colorectal lesion such as polyp, carcinoma, inflammatory bowel disease, diverticular disease).

Enquire about the presence of mucus or slime in the stool. If it is associated with blood, the most likely causes are inflammatory bowel disease or colorectal carcinoma. If mucus or slime occurs in isolation, irritable bowel syndrome may also be a cause.

Finally ask about other characteristics of the stool. For example:
- Reduced-calibre stools occur in low strictures.
- Fatty, floating, difficult to flush, offensive stools suggest steatorrhoea.
- Pellet-like or 'stringy' stools occur in diverticular disease or irritable bowel syndrome.

Medical history

A detailed history is essential, but previous surgical or medical problems may elucidate the cause of the change in bowel habit, for example:
- Previous colonic polyps, abdominal surgery.
- Thyroid disease.
- Malabsorption syndromes (e.g. pancreatitis).
- Diabetes mellitus (autonomic neuropathy).

Drug history

Many drugs can cause a change in bowel habit, for example:
- Constipation—opiates, anticholinergic agents, tricyclic antidepressants.
- Diarrhoea—thyroxine, laxative abuse, magnesium salts, broad-spectrum antibiotics (specifically consider pseudomembranous colitis).

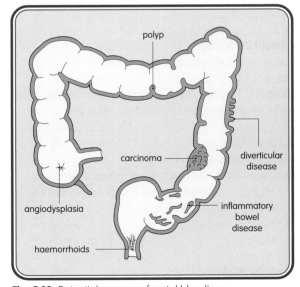

Fig. 5.12 Potential sources of rectal bleeding.

Family history

Some diseases causing a change in bowel habit have a genetic component, for example:

- Familial adenomatous polyposis.
- Inflammatory bowel disease.
- Carcinoma of the bowel.

Social history

Ask about foreign travel for amoebiasis, giardiasis, typhoid. If there is unexplained diarrhoea, consider the patient's risk factors for HIV infection.

DYSPHAGIA

Detailed history

Dysphagia refers to either difficulty in swallowing or pain on swallowing. Although the cause usually requires specific investigations (e.g. barium swallow, endoscopy, and biopsy), the history is important in directing these investigations. The main causes of dysphagia are indicated in Fig. 5.13.

What does the patient mean by dysphagia?

It is important to clarify exactly what patients mean when they say that they have difficulty in swallowing. It is not acceptable to write 'Patient complains of dysphagia' in the medical notes without clarification.

True dysphagia almost always indicates the presence of an organic lesion. It is important to distinguish dysphagia from the sensation of a lump or fullness in the throat (globus hystericus).

How bad is the dysphagia?

Try to assess the functional impact. Dysphagia often progresses from solid food to soft food and liquid. Ask the patient to describe exactly which foods cause difficulty. Ascertain whether there is complete obstruction (e.g. regurgitation immediately after attempting to swallow food, vomiting). Establish whether there has been any weight loss.

Duration and time course of symptoms

Ask patients how long they have had difficulty swallowing:

- Malignancy often presents over weeks or months and is typically progressive.
- An oesophageal ring may present over a similar time course, but produces a more intermittent pattern.
- Other causes may be present for years without any obvious systemic disturbance (e.g. globus hystericus).

Clues to underlying pathology

Specifically enquire about previous dyspepsia, proven peptic ulcer disease, or reflux. Ask about symptoms of heartburn such as acid taste in the mouth, retrosternal burning, relationship to posture. These symptoms suggest the presence of a benign oesophageal stricture.

Consider risk factors for oesophageal cancer such as:

- Cigarette smoking.
- Barrett's oesophagus.
- Old age.
- Heavy alcohol use.
- Significant weight loss.

Weight loss is a useful indicator of a serious underlying organic disorder and should always be asked about specifically.

Dysphagia to solid foods alone suggests a mechanical obstruction; dysphagia to solids and liquids early in the presentation suggests a neuromuscular cause.

Ask the patient where the food appears to get stuck. Symptoms such as difficulty initiating swallowing, coughing, choking, or nasal regurgitation suggest an oropharyngeal pathology. A sensation of food sticking after swallowing suggests an oesophageal lesion (Fig. 5.14).

Causes of dysphagia in the oesophagus	
Type of lesion	**Example**
obstruction within the lumen	carcinoma of the oesophagus; peptic stricture; foreign body; lower oesophageal ring
extrinsic compression of the oesophagus	massively enlarged left atrium; mediastinal lymphadenopathy
motility disorder of the oesophagus	achalasia of the oesophagus; oesophageal spasm; scleroderma; Chagas' disease; diabetic autonomic neuropathy

Fig. 5.13 Causes of dysphagia in the oesophagus.

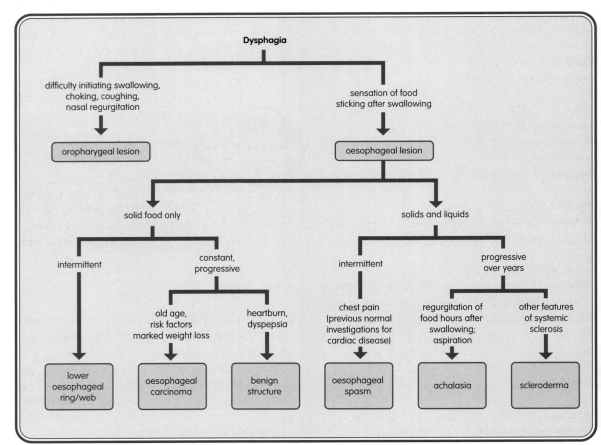

Fig. 5.14 Features from the history to aid the differential diagnosis of dysphagia.

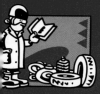

6. Presenting Problems: Renal Tract

Presenting complaint

Patients may present in various ways and these include the following:

- With symptoms directly referable to the renal tract (relatively rare presentation) (e.g. with haematuria, loin pain).
- With the consequences of renal failure (e.g. oedema, uraemic symptoms, hypertension).
- As an incidental finding from laboratory investigation (e.g. urinalysis, biochemical profile from investigation of other disease).
- Change in urine output.

Detailed history

Ask specifically about uraemic symptoms as these may indicate the need for haemodialysis. Ask about:

- Nausea, vomiting.
- Anorexia.
- Malaise, lethargy.
- Pruritus.
- Hiccupping.

Note that many of these symptoms are non-specific.

Specifically enquire about symptoms referable to the urinary tract as these may indicate the aetiology of renal dysfunction, for example:

- Prostatism—may suggest outflow obstruction.
- Haematuria—enquire specifically about the colour if haematuria is present (often described as 'like coca cola' in glomerulonephritis; bright red usually implies lower urinary tract bleeding).
- Dysuria, frequency (may suggest infective aetiology).
- Oliguria or anuria (may suggest prerenal disease or severe renal failure).
- 'Frothy urine' (e.g. in nephrotic states due to high protein content).

Complications of renal failure

These may be present, for example:

- Peripheral oedema.
- Hypertension.
- Dyspnoea due to pulmonary oedema.

Duration of disease

It is important to try to ascertain the duration of renal disease, as recent damage is much more amenable to specific treatment. It is not uncommon for a patient to have chronic renal failure and to be completely asymptomatic.

It is often difficult to elicit the duration of the disease as often the symptoms begin insidiously and are usually very non-specific. Clues may be obtained by asking specifically about, for example, change in weight or fatigue. "When did you last feel completely well?" "When could you last walk a mile?" This may date the onset of renal failure, but usually renal pathology remains clinically silent until decompensation occurs or it is discovered incidentally. However, a meticulous history may help date the original renal insult in different circumstances.

Hospitalized patients

Most cases of acute renal failure occur in hospital. Create a flow chart of the blood results (especially biochemical profile) dating back to the decline in renal function. It is often possible to identify within one or two days when the creatinine started to rise. At this point, focus on events occurring to the patient that might have provided a critical insult to the kidneys (e.g. period of hypotension or dehydration, toxic levels of aminoglycosides, coexisting infection).

New referral from the community

Almost invariably, there is less immediate information to chart, but it is still essential to obtain historical records of previous renal function. Clues may be obtained from various sources (e.g. previous blood test results, results of urinalysis for women who have previously been pregnant).

Past medical history

As the causes of renal failure are numerous, an extremely detailed past medical history is essential. In particular consider:

- Diabetes mellitus—duration, and presence of neuropathy or retinopathy, which are almost invariably associated with diabetic nephropathy.
- Hypertension—did it predate or postdate renal dysfunction?
- Risk factors for renovascular disease—for example, claudication, aortic aneurysm, ischaemic heart disease, hypercholesterolaemia.
- Childhood enuresis or frequent urinary tract infections suggesting reflux nephropathy.
- Renal stones or colic.
- Autoimmune diseases—for example, systemic lupus erythematosus (SLE), rheumatoid arthritis, scleroderma.
- Jaundice—for example, hepatitis B, C-associated glomerulopathy, leptospirosis, hepatorenal syndrome.
- Recent infections—for example, postinfectious glomerulonephritis (rare), presentation of IgA nephropathy with haematuria following a sore throat.

Drug history

Again, a detailed drug history is essential. Very often, drugs have precipitated the renal failure. Remember to ask about over-the-counter (OTC) medication and herbal remedies.

Drugs may precipitate renal failure by various mechanisms (Fig. 6.1).

Other drugs must be used with caution in renal failure. For example:

- Renally excreted drugs (aminoglycosides).
- If there is an accumulation of metabolites due to failure of clearance (opiates).

Family history

Consider inherited conditions (e.g. polycystic kidneys, Alport's syndrome).

Social history

It is essential to obtain as much background information as possible to assess normal functional capacity. In addition, consider whether the patient's lifestyle may have contributed to the renal failure, for example:

- Cigarette smoking (renovascular disease).
- Alcohol (hepatorenal disease).
- Risk factors for HIV and hepatitis B,C (glomerulonephritis, hepatorenal disease).
- Travel and ethnic origin—many forms of

Mechanisms of drug-induced renal dysfunction	
Pathology	**Drugs**
decreased renal perfusion	diuretics* (hypovolaemia); NSAIDs* (also cause interstitial nephritis, hyperkalaemia, and rarely papillary necrosis)
decreased glomerular filtration pressure	ACE inhibitors*
nephrotic syndrome	gold; penicillamine
acute tubular necrosis	aminoglycosides* (especially if toxic drug levels); antibiotics (e.g. cephalosporins); contrast agents (especially in diabetics); chemotherapy (e.g. cisplatin)
interstitial nephritis	NSAIDs*, antibiotics* (e.g. penicillin, sulphonamides)
renal stones	cytotoxic agents (especially in lymphoma)
electrolyte disturbances	diuretics* (especially hypokalaemia); renal tubular acidosis (acetazolamide) inappropriate ADH secretion (carbamazepine, chlorpropamide); hyperkalaemia (NSAIDs, ACE inhibitors, diuretics acting on distal tubule)
retroperitoneal fibrosis	methysergide

Fig. 6.1 Mechanisms of drug-induced renal dysfunction. * indicates the more commonly implicated drugs. (ACE, angiotensin-converting enzyme; ADH, antidiuretic hormone; NSAID, non-steroidal anti-inflammatory drug.)

glomerulonephritis demonstrate great geographical variation (e.g. IgA nephropathy is more common in Caucasians, SLE is more common in Afro-Caribbeans).

Review of systems enquiry

Vital information may be omitted if a systems enquiry is not performed. In particular, consider:

- Symptoms suggestive of autoimmune aetiology—skin rash, arthralgia, myalgia, alopecia, early morning stiffness.
- Haemoptysis—pulmonary vasculitis (rare).
- Fevers—any infective or inflammatory disease.
- Risk factors for ischaemic heart disease.

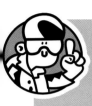

It is often the most meticulous and tenacious historian who is rewarded when clerking patients with renal failure. Although the pathological diagnosis is usually made by imaging, laboratory, and histological investigations, there are numerous causes of renal failure, and focused investigation begins with the history.

CHRONIC RENAL FAILURE

Presenting complaint

It is assumed that the patient will already be on dialysis or is being reviewed in the predialysis clinic and that the cause of renal disease has already been investigated (see previous section).

Detailed history
Dialysis

Assess symptoms indicative of inadequate dialysis or need to commence dialysis such as:

- Anorexia.
- Nausea, vomiting.
- Fatigue, malaise.
- Pruritus.
- Confusion, drowsiness.

Although many of these symptoms are non-specific, if no other cause is found, assume that they represent uraemia.

Dialysis-related problems

Dialysis is associated with a number of specific problems or issues, which need to be considered whether the form of dialysis is peritoneal dialysis or haemodialysis. Review the mechanics and complications of dialysis (Fig. 6.2).

Features of peritoneal dialysis and haemodialysis to elicit from the history		
Parameter	Peritoneal dialysis	Haemodialysis
mode of dialysis	continuous ambulatory peritoneal dialysis (CAPD); automated peritoneal dialysis (APD)	hospital haemodialysis; home haemodialysis
dialysis dose	number and type of bags (e.g. 'light/heavy'); volume of fluid (typically 2 L)	hours on dialysis; frequency (typically 4 hours three times weekly)
access	PD exit site	arteriovenous (AV) fistula; temporary catheter (e.g. 'vascath'); AV shunt
complications of dialysis	peritonitis; exit site and tunnel infections	dialysis disequilibrium; hypotensive episodes; difficulty needling fistula; exit site infections: vascular stenosis

Fig. 6.2 Features of peritoneal dialysis (PD) and haemodialysis (HD).

Fluid balance

There are many common problems of chronic renal failure and these should always be addressed. Review fluid balance as this is central to the management. It is essential to ask about the following:

- Does the patient have a target 'dry' weight? Fluctuations from this weight in the short term usually indicate fluid shifts.
- Urine output and daily fluid restriction, which is usually 500 mL more than daily urine output.
- Interdialytic weight gains. Large gains may indicate poor compliance and understanding of self-management.

Anaemia

Review symptoms (e.g. dyspnoea, lethargy, decreased exercise tolerance). Many patients will be receiving recombinant erythropoietin. Always specifically enquire about and record:

- The dose.
- Side effects (e.g. hypertension, hyperkalaemia).
- Reasons for lack of response to erythropoietin (e.g. iron deficiency, intercurrent infection, hyperparathyroidism).

Renal osteodystrophy

Renal osteodystrophy is a common problem of chronic renal failure and should be explored. From the notes and patient account, review the following factors:

- Calcium and phosphate balance.
- Diet.
- Calcium carbonate dose.
- Biochemical evidence for hyperparathyroidism.

Transplant status

Review plans for discharging the patient from this form of dialysis. In particular, consider (at every visit) the appropriateness for transplantation:

- Taking into account the patient's wishes and education.
- Reviewing intercurrent medical issues that may preclude transplantation—for example, age, infection, malignancy, severe vascular disease, untreated ischaemic heart disease, active peptic ulceration.

Blood pressure control

Review the documentary evidence of blood pressure measurements, for example from dialysis charts or recordings made at home (before erythropoietin dosing) or by the general practitioner.

Past medical history

This is usually well known. Do not forget the original cause of the renal failure!

Drug history

A meticulous drug history is essential. Very often, the patient will have a long list of medication. Enquire specifically about:

- Antihypertensive agents.
- Erythropoietin (see above).
- Phosphate binders and vitamin D.
- Iron supplements.
- OTC medication.

Consider drugs to be used with caution in renal failure (see 'Acute renal failure', p. 48).

Social history

A detailed assessment should be made, especially in the predialysis patient, when considering whether dialysis would be appropriate and, if so, which form.

If considering haemodialysis:
- Will transport be needed to the hospital?
- Does the patient have motivation and space at home, and a partner for home haemodialysis ?

If considering continuous ambulatory peritoneal dialysis (CAPD), the following questions should be asked:
- Does the patient have space at home to store boxes containing peritoneal dialysis fluid?
- Does the patient have the manual dexterity needed to change bags?
- Does the patient have the motivation and intelligence to manage the care so that there is not an undue risk for developing peritonitis or exit site infections?
- Is the patient too obese?

Review the patient's nutrition and diet. This is often specialized, and referral to a renal dietician is indicated.

Review of systems enquiry

This is particularly important, as often these patients are multisymptomatic and renal failure is associated with so many other diseases (e.g. ischaemic heart disease, arthritis, gastrointestinal bleeding).

Chronic renal failure results in multisystem dysfunction. Assessment needs to be detailed. It is pointless to rush. Always allow enough time.

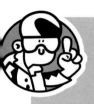

In predialysis patients check that adequate plans have been made for the initiation of dialysis so that the transition can be as smooth as possible. Consider patient education, mode of intended dialysis, access for dialysis, and estimated time to dialysis initiation.

- "Are there any clots in your urine?"
- "Is your urine bright red or stained like Ribena?"
- "Does your urine appear cloudy or like cola?" (glomerulonephritis).

The timing of blood during the urinary stream may provide a clue to the origin of bleeding. For example:
- Bleeding at the start of the urinary stream suggests a urethral lesion.
- Bleeding through the whole stream suggests a source in the bladder or higher in the urinary tract.
- Bleeding at the end of the urinary stream suggests a source in the lower bladder.

Associated urinary symptoms

Other symptoms referable to the urinary tract often provide useful clues to the cause of haematuria. Specifically ask about:
- Dysuria and frequency with small quantities of urine—urinary tract infection.
- Dysuria and frequency in association with fever and loin pain—suggests pyelonephritis.
- Colicky loin pain—indicative of renal stones.
- Symptoms of renal disease such as ankle swelling or uraemic symptoms (see p. 47).
- Terminal dribbling, hesitancy, and poor stream—common in prostatic obstruction.

HAEMATURIA

Detailed history

Haematuria is a common symptom and may be due to a wide variety of pathologies (Fig. 6.3).

Take a full history of the presenting symptom.

Ascertain that true haematuria is present

Some patients with uterine bleeding mistakenly believe that they have haematuria.

Duration

Note whether the haematuria is an acute presentation or has been present for many years or months.

Nature

Haematuria is an alarming symptom and usually causes patients to consult their doctor. A small amount of blood produces visible discolouration of the urine. Try to establish how much blood is present in the urine. It may be helpful to ask:

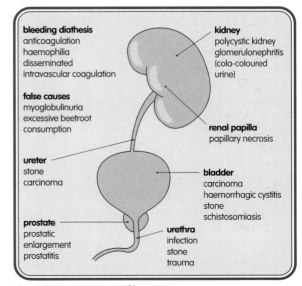

Fig. 6.3 Some causes of haematuria.

bleeding diathesis
anticoagulation
haemophilia
disseminated intravascular coagulation

false causes
myoglobulinuria
excessive beetroot consumption

ureter
stone
carcinoma

prostate
prostatic enlargement
prostatitis

kidney
polycystic kidney
glomerulonephritis (cola-coloured urine)

renal papilla
papillary necrosis

bladder
carcinoma
haemorrhagic cystitis
stone
schistosomiasis

urethra
infection
stone
trauma

Past medical history

A detailed past medical history is important. In particular, ask about:

- Previous renal disease.
- Abdominal trauma (e.g. renal capsular tear).
- Renal stones or previous episodes of colic.
- Previous cystoscopies.
- Prostatectomy (in men).
- Sickle-cell anaemia (papillary necrosis).

Drug history

Some drugs may aggravate or cause haematuria. For example:

- Cyclophosphamide (haemorrhagic cystitis, carcinoma of the bladder).
- Warfarin (bleeding diathesis).
- Analgesic abuse (papillary necrosis).

Family history

Many renal diseases have a familial tendency. For example:

- Alport's syndrome (X-linked recessive). Ask about deafness.
- IgA nephropathy. Ask about the relationship of macroscopic haematuria to infections.
- Polycystic kidney disease (adult variety is autosomal dominant).
- Sickle-cell anaemia.

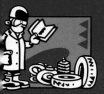

7. Presenting Problems: Nervous System

THE UNCONSCIOUS PATIENT

Detailed history

Paradoxically, the history is especially important in the evaluation of the unconscious patient, even if it does not come from the patient. Obtain the history from relatives or friends, the ambulance crew, and police, if appropriate. Try to establish the following.

Time of onset of unconsciousness

Who found the patient unconscious, and when? When was the patient last seen conscious? Where was the patient found?

Duration of illness preceding unconsciousness

Had the patient been well before being found unconscious? Was the illness sudden, subacute, or chronic?

Nature of the preceding illness

It is helpful to consider the differential diagnosis, so that questions can be more focused (Fig. 7.1).

Past medical history

Obtain a full history. There may have been previous episodes. Enquire specifically about:
- Diabetes mellitus (hypoglycaemia, hyperglycaemic coma).
- Risk factors for cerebrovascular disease (stroke).
- Liver failure.
- Head trauma—no matter how mild and how much in the past; a subdural haematoma may be preceded by a history of a trivial head injury, especially in the elderly.
- Epilepsy and other neurological disorders.
- Renal failure.
- Preceding headaches—for example, meningitis, intracranial mass lesion, subarachnoid haemorrhage.
- Vomiting.

Drug history

Consider all drugs that may depress the conscious level if taken in therapeutic or toxic amounts. Remember to ask about analgesic agents and psychotropic medication.

Social history

This is particularly important, especially in younger patients. Ask specifically about:
- Alcohol (very important).
- Drugs of abuse (very important).
- Possible reasons for deliberate self-harm.
- Risk factors for HIV infection (if appropriate).

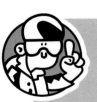

Detailed history taking often needs to be deferred until appropriate resuscitation or stabilization has been carried out.

Do not underestimate the importance of the history, even if the patient cannot provide one directly. The differential diagnosis is broad, but can usually be narrowed down with the aid of a well-taken history.

Clues from the history on the underlying cause of unconsciousness	
Description	**Indications**
vascular* subarachnoid haemorrhage*	preceding headache; sudden onset; often young adult; may have had 'herald bleed'
intracerebral bleed*, massive infarction*, brainstem stroke *	risk factors for cerebrovascular disease (hypertension, diabetes mellitus (DM), ischaemic heart disease, age, family history, etc.)
metabolic* DM*	hyperosmolar coma (type II DM); diabetic ketoacidosis (type I—may be presenting feature of disease); hypoglycaemia
drugs and toxins*	alcohol*; sedative drugs (opiates, benzodiazepines, barbiturates, etc.)
hypoxia, hyponatraemia, hypothyroidism*, uraemia, hepatic encephalopathy	often present non-specifically
sepsis generalized, meningoencephalitis, brain abscess	usually preceding illness; ask about rash, photophobia, fevers, headache, vomiting, etc.
subdural*/extradural haematoma	may be history of trauma (often absent)
postictal	may find bottle of anti-epileptic tablets
intracranial mass lesion	ask about features of raised intracranial pressure (e.g. increasing morning headache, vomiting, developing focal neurological problems)
factitious/hysteria	often unusual presentation; past psychiatric history

Fig. 7.1 Clues from the history on the underlying cause of unconsciousness. * indicates the more common causes.

BLACKOUTS

Detailed history

A common problem for admitting medical teams is the investigation of a patient who has had a blackout. The history is central to the diagnosis. Follow the usual systematic approach to investigate circumstances of the blackout. It is helpful to consider the differential diagnosis of blackouts (Fig. 7.2)

Investigate the episode chronologically. Find out what the patient was doing immediately before blacking out, whether the patient had any warning symptoms, and how the patient felt immediately after regaining consciousness (Fig. 7.3).

Did anyone witness the episode?

This is probably the most useful piece of information. If so, ask specifically about:

- How long the blackout lasted (seconds, minutes, or hours).
- What was the patient doing during the episode (e.g. lying still, shaking, appearing confused, purposeful movements).
- The presence of any tongue biting, shaking, or incontinence to suggest an epileptic fit.
- Did anyone feel the pulse either during or immediately after the blackout? A normal pulse during the blackout would exclude an arrhythmia.

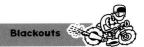

Differential diagnosis of blackouts

epilepsy*

decreased cerebral perfusion
vasovagal episode*; cardiac disturbances* (e.g. arrhythmia, aortic stenosis, ischaemia); postural hypotension*; TIA (especially in posterior circulation); micturition syncope (decreased venous return during breath holding); cough syncope (decreased venous return); carotid sinus hypersensitivity

metabolic disturbances
hypoglycaemia; hypocalcaemia

psychological
panic attacks*; hyperventilation*; factitious

drugs
alcohol*; recreational drugs of abuse; prescribed medication (e.g. decreased threshold for epileptic fit, sedative, β-blockers provoking profound bradycardia, etc.)

Fig. 7.2 Differential diagnosis of blackouts. * indicates the more common causes. (TIA, transient ischaemic attack.)

Clues from the history on the underlying pathology responsible for an episode of loss of consciousness

Clues from the history	Possible underlying cause of blackout
What were you doing immediately before blacking out? standing up quickly turning head sharply vigorous exertion trauma completely at rest standing still in hot environment	postural hypotension cervical spondylosis (occlusion of vertebral artery) aortic stenosis; ischaemic heart disease subdural haematoma; extradural haematoma; contusion injury arrhythmia; cerebrovascular disease, etc. vasovagal
Did you have any warning that you were going to blackout? aura palpitations, chest pain lightheadedness sweating, hunger	epileptic fit cardiogenic; panic attack vasovagal, etc. hypoglycaemia

Fig. 7.3 Clues from the history on the underlying pathology responsible for an episode of loss of consciousness.

Try to establish whether the episode was a true syncopal attack (loss of conciousness and motor tone) or just a period of lightheadedness. Very often people say that they have blacked out when they do not completely lose consciousness: ask for example "Did you lose any time?"

Enquire about the immediate period following recovery of consciousness. Symptoms at this stage may give clues to the precipitating event, for example:
- Immediate recovery—vasovagal.
- Post-ictal.

- Weakness—Todd's paralysis, transient ischaemic attack (TIA).

Past medical history

Ask about previous blackouts and investigations performed. Consider clues from the past history that may increase the probability of certain underlying problems, for example:
- Risk factors for epilepsy—for example, head injury, cerebrovascular disease, meningitis.
- Cardiac diseases.

- Diabetes mellitus—enquire about diabetic control and previous episodes of hypoglycaemia.

Drug history
A full drug history is essential. In particular, consider:
- Recent changes to prescribed drugs.
- Negative chronotropic and inotropic agents (e.g. β-blockers).
- Drugs likely to cause arrhythmias (e.g. tricyclic antidepressants, theophylline).
- Insulin (hypoglycaemia).
- Antihypertensive agents (postural hypotension).
- Glyceryl trinitrate (GTN) syncope.
- Illicit drug use

Social history
Investigate whether the home environment is safe for someone who may black out unexpectedly (e.g. are there any carers at home?). The patient's lifestyle may suggest underlying risks for a blackout (e.g. alcohol consumption, unusual stresses at home or work, social life).

Ask about driving. Should the Driver and Vehicle Licensing Authority (DVLA) be informed of this episode?

Review of systems enquiry
Blackouts may result from a wide range of pathologies, so a review of systems may reveal unexpected pathology. Focus on the cardiovascular, neurological, metabolic, and locomotor systems.

The key to diagnosing the cause of a blackout is a well-taken history. The most useful information comes from an eyewitness account.

HEADACHE

Detailed history
Consider the following common causes of single and recurrent headaches:
- Tension headache (by far the most common).
- Migraine (common).

- Hangover (apparent from the history).
- Subarachnoid haemorrhage (rare, but consider for any sudden-onset headache).
- Meningitis, encephalitis.
- Raised intracranial pressure (e.g. tumour, hydrocephalus).
- Temporal arteritis.

Obtain a detailed history about the frequency of headaches: for example, recurrent heaches are typically tension headaches or migraine, while a headache every morning can be due to raised intracranial pressure associated with a tumour.

Obtain information about the onset, nature, and location of headache. It is often possible to identify the cause of a headache from these parameters (Figs 7.4 and 7.5).

For any new-onset headache, always ask specifically about photophobia, neck stiffness, rash, fever, and vomiting.

Past medical history
Ask specifically about previous malignancy if raised intracranial pressure is suspected.

Drug history
Ask about medication taken to relieve symptoms and efficacy. It is often hard to assess the severity of headache as people can rarely give a quantitative description. It may be worth asking "If 0 is no pain, and 10 is the worst headache you have ever had, what score would you give this pain?" Ask girls and women about the use of oral contraceptives (may provoke or worsen migraine, particularly in the pill-free week).

Social history
For recurrent headaches, it is essential to ask about stresses, for example at home and work, that may be provoking chronic non-specific headaches. The patient's alcohol history is also relevant.

Features of different types of headache	
Headache	**Characteristics**
tension headache	most common recurrent headache, typically described as 'throbbing', 'pressure', etc.; often identifiable precipitating factor (e.g. stress, depression)
migraine	common cause of recurrent headache; usually presents in young adults; prodrome—often visual (e.g. scotomata, teichopsia), tingling, etc.; headache—often starts unilaterally; associated symptoms (e.g. nausea, vomiting, photophobia, etc.)
subarachnoid haemorrhage	may have had 'herald bleed' with milder 'subclinical' episodes; typically sudden onset 'like a hammer hitting the back of my head'; may have associated neurological deficit or decreased level of consciousness
hangover	preceding alcohol consumption; associated nausea
meningitis	photophobia; neck stiffness; fever; rash
raised intracranial pressure	usually subacute onset; relentless; present on waking; aggravated by coughing, sneezing, stooping; associated nausea.
temporal arteritis	pain over superficial temporal arteries, especially on touching area (e.g. combing hair); may have associated malaise, proximal muscle weakness, and stiffness, and visual loss; usually older than 60 years

Fig. 7.4 Features of different types of headache.

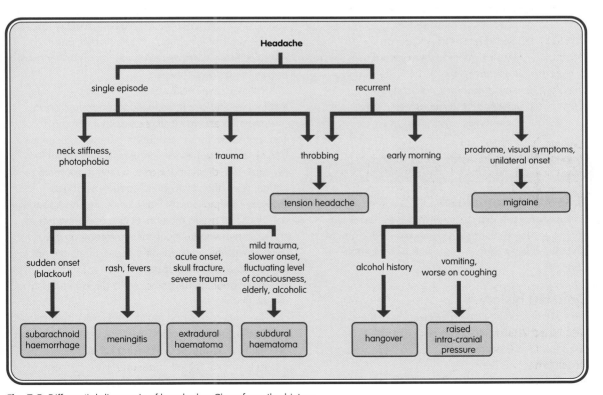

Fig. 7.5 Differential diagnosis of headache. Clues from the history.

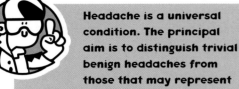

Headache is a universal condition. The principal aim is to distinguish trivial benign headaches from those that may represent serious underlying pathology needing further investigation so that appropriate reassurance can be given and unnecessary investigation avoided (especially in the case of the somatising patient).

Always consider headaches representing serious disease. Alarm words may include:
- Scalp tenderness, proximal limb stiffness—temporal arteritis.
- Rash, fever, photophobia, neck stiffness—meningitis.
- Sudden-onset occipital headache—subarachnoid haemorrhage.
- Early morning headache, nausea—raised intracranial pressure.

EPILEPTIC FIT

Presenting complaint

Epilepsy may present as an unwitnessed blackout (single or recurrent) or as an eyewitness account of a fit. More rarely it may present with behavioural changes.

Detailed history

Start with the patient's own recollection of the event, recording the following chronologically.

Prodrome

Ask: "Did you have any warning that you were going to black out?" Typical auras include complex mental states, emotions, or hallucinations (e.g. smell, taste, vision). They often follow a predictable course for the individual patient.

Seizure

Ask: "Tell me what you remember about the attack." "Did you black out and lose consciousness?"

The answers to these questions may help distinguish between generalized and partial seizures. If the patient was conscious during the episode, ask him or her to describe exactly what happened. If the patient has experienced a partial seizure, the symptoms are often characteristic of the site of epileptic focus, for example:
- Jacksonian motor seizures.
- Temporal lobe epilepsy (déjà vu, jamais vu, hallucinations of smell or taste, etc.).

It is usually possible to distinguish partial seizures, generalized seizures, and partial seizures with secondary generalization.

Postictal period

Ask: "How did you feel when you came around?" It is usual to experience a headache, 'muzziness', lethargy, confusion, and non-specific malaise. A focal weakness may be present for up to 24 hours (Todd's paralysis). Ask specifically whether the patient bit his or her tongue or had urinary incontinence.

Obtain an eyewitness account if possible. This is invaluable, and can provide diagnostic information.

If the episode was a single blackout, the most common difficulty is distinguishing between epilepsy and syncope. Look for an identifiable precipitant for syncope (e.g. emotional stress, prolonged standing, cough, micturition syncope). Gradual onset and recovery, and pallor and flaccidity during the episode are all characteristic features of syncope. Beware! A convulsion or urinary incontinence rarely can occur during syncopal episodes so these features are not pathognomonic of epilepsy.

On the basis of the history, try to decide on the type of epilepsy (Fig. 7.6).

If the patient has had multiple fits, ask about seizure control (i.e. frequency of fits, duration of fits). Ask about precipitating factors (e.g. flickering lights).

Past medical history

Consider possible underlying causes of fits (Fig. 7.7).

Drug history

Ask about drugs used to control epilepsy, and their side effects (e.g. phenytoin, sodium valproate, carbamazepine). Ask specifically about symptoms suggestive of overdose (e.g. drowsiness, ataxia, slurred speech). Review compliance, especially if

Historical features of different types of epilepsy	
generalized seizures	
tonic–clonic seizure (grand mal fit)*	most commonly perceived form of epilepsy— 'convulsions'
absence seizures (petit mal)*	especially in childhood; brief (few seconds) loss of consciousness; no fall; no convulsion
myoclonic seizures	especially in childhood; usually symmetrical
tonic seizures	especially in childhood; loss of consciousness; usually underlying organic brain disease
akinetic seizures	no prodrome ('drop attacks')
partial seizures	
simple partial seizures*	remains fully conscious during attack (e.g. jacksonian fit)
complex partial seizures*	originates in the temporal lobe; often complex sensory hallucinations, déja vu, jamais vu, lip smacking, chewing, behavioural disturbances; etc.
partial seizure with secondary generalization*	as above, but progresses to tonic-clonic seizure

Fig. 7.6 The history often reveals the type of epilepsy. * indicates the more common causes.

Underlying pathology causing epileptic fits

cerebrovascular disease*
most common cause in older age group; risk factors (e.g. hypertension, smoking, ischaemic heart disease, diabetes mellitus, etc.)

alcohol and drug withdrawal*

drugs*
for example tricyclic antidepressants, phenothiazines, amphetamines, etc.

head injury and neurosurgery

tumours

encephalitis

degenerative brain disease

metabolic disorders
for example hypoglycaemia, hyponatraemia, hypocalcaemia, uraemia, liver failure, etc.

fever
infants

Fig. 7.7 Underlying pathology responsible for epileptic fits can often be identified. * indicates the more common causes.

there is evidence of poor seizure control, and consider the need to check drug concentrations in plasma (phenytoin has a narrow therapeutic index).

Consider medication that may:

- Interact with anticonvulsants (e.g. oral contraceptives, warfarin).
- Lower the seizure threshold (e.g. phenothiazines, tricyclic antidepressants, amphetamines).

Family history

In younger patients, there is often a positive family history. Consider an inherited disorder (e.g. Tay–Sachs disease, ceroid lipofuscinoses, tuberous sclerosis).

Social history

There are multiple social issues surrounding epilepsy. Often, patients feel stigmatized and socially isolated. School performance is often poor. The reasons for this should be explored (e.g. poorly controlled seizures, drug intoxication, social isolation and bullying, underlying brain disease). Parents are often understandably overprotective. Consider sensible restrictions on activities for children while allowing a full social life (e.g. avoiding known precipitants such as strobe lighting at discos, bathing in a locked bathroom, dangerous sports such as rock climbing).

Review occupational problems (e.g. use of dangerous machinery, employers who do not understand the disease).

Consider the restrictions on driving. This may affect the decision to start withdrawing medication in patients with well-controlled disease if driving is particularly important to them. Consult the DVLA *Medical Aspects of Fitness to Drive* handbook for further information.

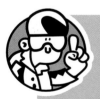

In common with many other neurological events, try to obtain a good eyewitness account of a typical episode as very often the patient is asymptomatic and has no physical signs on presentation to a doctor.

STROKE

Detailed history

Establish that the described event is a stroke. It is usually obvious from the history that a stroke has occurred.

A stroke is an acute focal neurological deficit due to a vascular lesion, lasting longer than 24 hours. A TIA is a focal neurological deficit due to a vascular lesion that resolves within 24 hours.

Onset

Obtain a chronological account of the onset and progression of neurological disability. Ask: "What were you doing immediately before this happened?" Typically strokes occur at rest, but patients may wake up to find that they cannot move a limb. The onset is typically immediate, but may evolve over a few hours—"One moment I was fine, and the next, I was unable to move my right arm".

Define the neurological disability, for example, ask: "What can't you do now that you could manage before this happened?" This is important because:

- It provides a baseline to assess recovery or subsequent deterioration.
- The anatomical site of the lesion can be identified. The neurological disability typically corresponds to the vascular territory of the occluded or haemorrhaging artery (Figs 7.8 and 7.9).
- It allows an assessment of whether the event is likely to be a stroke or a TIA and any evidence of recovery between the onset and presentation.

Past medical history

Consider the possible aetiology of the stroke as this will affect subsequent management (Fig. 7.10). Ask specifically about previous TIAs, amaurosis fugax, peripheral vascular disease (PVD).

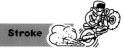
Neurological deficits due to lesions in different vascular territories	
Vascular territory	**Clinical pattern**
anterior cerebral artery	contralateral hemiplegia; predominant leg weakness; disturbance of micturition; apraxia
middle cerebral artery (internal carotid artery)	most common; contralateral hemiplegia with predominant upper limb weakness and facial weakness; dysphasia; hemianopia
posterior circulation	vertigo; diplopia; ataxia; nystagmus; often prominent headache; may have hemiplegia affecting opposite side to cranial nerve lesions
lacunar infarcts	may be asymptomatic; usually cause mild stroke, which may be limited to pure motor or sensory disturbance, sudden dysarthria, etc.

Fig. 7.8 Features of neurological deficits due to lesions in different vascular territories.

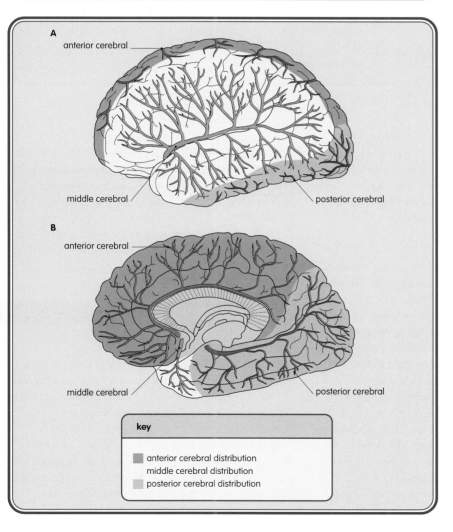

A

anterior cerebral

middle cerebral

posterior cerebral

B

anterior cerebral

middle cerebral

posterior cerebral

key

▪ anterior cerebral distribution
▫ middle cerebral distribution
▪ posterior cerebral distribution

Fig. 7.9 The vascular territories of the main cerebral arteries. (A) Lateral view of a cerebral hemisphere. (B) Sagittal section through the cerebral hemispheres

Common causes of stroke	
Pathology	**Features in the history**
ischaemic stroke*—thrombosis*, embolism*	by far the most common; ischaemic heart disease, diabetes mellitus, hypertension, smoking, valvular heart disease (especially mitral stenosis/prosthetic heart valve), atrial fibrillation, family history, older age; hyperviscosity (e.g. polycythaemia, Waldenstrom's macroglobulinaemia)
cerebral haemorrhage*	common; as above, but hypertension is often pronounced; headache is often a prominent feature as is a disturbed level of consciousness
extradural haematoma	severe head injury
subdural haematoma	history of head injury (often mild); alcoholic; old age
subarachnoid haemorrhage	'herald bleeds', sudden-onset headache; loss of consciousness common; meningism
vasculitis	giant cell arteritis, systemic lupus erythematosus (SLE), Wegener's granulomatosis, sarcoidosis, etc. (consider features of above diseases)
infections	syphilis, infective endocarditis (rare)

Fig. 7.10 Common causes of stroke. * indicates the more common causes.

Drug history

Ask specifically about warfarin, aspirin, and heparin if an intracranial bleed is suspected. Reviewing the list of medication often highlights a risk factor that the patient or his or her relatives may have forgotten.

Social history

An extremely detailed social assessment is necessary to ascertain if and when the patient can be discharged home. Remember that discharge planning should begin at the point of admission to hospital.

The diagnosis of stroke is usually apparent on presentation, but an attempt should be made to define its aetiology and severity. At present, for the vast majority of patients presenting with stroke, there is little specific medical therapy that has been demonstrated to significantly limit subsequent neurological deficit. The bulk of treatment will be supportive to aid rehabilitation. This relies upon an adequate initial assessment and the detailed social history is essential for coordinating the various members of the multidisciplinary team (e.g. physiotherapist, occupational therapist, social worker, dietician, speech therapist).

When stroke is diagnosed, coordinate all members of the multidisciplinary team as soon as possible. Discharge planning should begin on admission to hospital.

'OFF LEGS'

Detailed history

Elderly people often present in a non-specific manner with difficulty functioning at home with their normal day to day activities. The ability to compensate for relatively minor physiological derangements is impaired in the elderly. The differential diagnosis is enormous, and represents one of the greatest challenges in history taking. Consider some of the more common underlying disorders listed below that may present non-specifically as confusion or inability to cope at home (the more common are denoted with an asterisk):

- Infection* (e.g. urinary tract infection*, chest infection).
- Drugs*—very common (e.g. diuretics causing electrolyte disturbances, sedatives, antihypertensives).
- Metabolic—for example hypothyroidism*, hyperthyroidism, diabetes mellitus (new presentation or established disease), electrolyte disturbances* (e.g. hyponatraemia, hypernatraemia, hypercalcaemia), dehydration.
- Neurological (e.g. dementia*, Parkinson's disease, subdural haematoma*).
- Cardiovascular—for example cerebrovascular disease*, myocardial infarction* (e.g. heart failure*, hypotension*), arrhythmias* (especially atrial fibrillation*).
- Haematological (e.g. anaemia due to peptic ulceration, bowel cancer, vitamin B_{12} or folate deficiency).
- Liver disease.
- Psychiatric (e.g. depression*).

Much of the medical dictionary can be added to this list, including apparently mundane conditions (e.g. urinary retention, constipation).

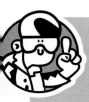

Often the history from the patient is vague or uninformative. A detailed history from friends, family, or other carers is invaluable.

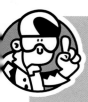

Elderly patients often present with multiple patholgies. Once one problem is identified, it is still important to search for others.

Try to obtain a chronological, systematic history in the usual way, focusing on:
- Time course.
- Rate of decline (e.g. a sudden decline over minutes may suggest of a vascular event; acute decline over hours or days may suggest an infective or metabolic disorder; a chronic decline may be due to dementia).
- Pattern of dysfunction (e.g. stepwise deterioration, sudden decline, relapsing and remitting).
- Functional skills. Ask "What does he (or she) have difficulty doing now that he (or she) could manage last week?"

Past medical history

A detailed past medical history should be obtained. The dysfunctional state may result from deterioration of a pre-existing condition or a new event superimposed on a pathological process. In particular ask about:
- Ischaemic heart disease and cerebrovascular disease (including risk factors).
- Diabetes mellitus.
- Psychiatric disorders (dementia, depression).
- Malignancy.

Drug history

The drug history is particularly important. Often the carer may not be aware of the detailed past medical history and the patient may not be in a state to provide one, so a look at the patient's medication may offer clues about pre-existing conditions. Alternatively, the drugs often contribute to the presentation. Concentrate on:
- Newly prescribed medication—why? When? Effect?
- Psychotropic medication (e.g. sleeping tablets, antidepressants).
- Antihypertensive medication (especially if newly prescribed).
- Drugs that may cause electrolyte derangement (e.g. diuretics).

Social history

The social history is central to a full assessment. It is important to understand the normal pattern of daily activities and how they are normally negotiated (e.g. dressing, bathing, cooking, toileting, shopping, managing medication, social interaction).

Assess the social support usually provided, and the possibility that this could be improved (e.g. family, friends, home help, meals on wheels, district nurse, previous social worker involvement).

Consider other factors in the patient's lifestyle that may have contributed to decompensation, for example:

- Alcohol—often a contributory factor in declining social functioning.
- Smoking history—may highlight risk factors (e.g. for cardiovascular disease, chest disease, malignancy).
- Diet and nutrition—often inadequate in elderly patients.

Elderly patients often present in a non-specific manner with an inability to cope in their home environment. This is an inadequate diagnosis and a thorough assessment should be made to elucidate the reason(s) behind this. Usually there are multiple pathologies. Try to diagnose each individual problem and consider which ones are active and which are responsible for the current presentation. Do not ignore apparently trivial illnesses! Review the home circumstances in detail and consider whether the home is safe in the short term or a more detailed assessment is needed (e.g. by occupational therapists and social workers).

Review of systems enquiry

There are few circumstances when it is more important to perform a thorough review of systems enquiry. Inability of elderly people to cope in their home environment is usually due to the interaction of multiple pathologies reaching a critical level and resulting in decompensation. If adequate time is allowed, it usually becomes apparent that the patient was polysymptomatic from different systems before this presentation. For example, an elderly man may have:

- Osteoarthritis affecting his hips and limiting mobility.
- Early Alzheimer's dementia.
- A peptic ulcer resulting in iron-deficiency anaemia.
- Urinary retention due to prostatism.
- Recently prescribed tricyclic antidepressant.

It is sometimes difficult to distinguish symptoms relevant to the current presentation, but that is part of the skill and fun of good history taking!

Spend time establishing the patient's baseline function so that realistic targets for therapy can be set.

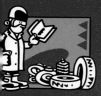

8. Presenting Problems: Psychiatric

DRUG OVERDOSE

Detailed history

There is a wide spectrum of patients who present with a drug overdose. Some have had a genuine desire to commit suicide, but many are impulsive or manipulative acts. Whatever the motivation of the patient, the initial history is often difficult to elicit. The first priority is to establish whether any specific therapeutic measures are needed, and to institute these. If necessary, a more detailed history can be taken in a less stressful environment at a later stage.

Establish the medication taken and dosage consumed

Try to obtain information about the medication taken, from either the patient or a witness. The patient may volunteer this information, but is often reluctant. Ask the witness whether anyone in the household has prescribed medication or any pill bottles were found close to the patient. Fig. 8.1 lists the top ten agents responsible for fatal self-poisoning.

Top ten agents responsible for fatal self-poisoning (OPCS mortality statistics)	
Agent	**Number of deaths/year**
1. carbon monoxide	976
2. co-proxamol	125
3. dothiepin	69
4. paracetamol	64
5. amitriptyline	45
6. temazepam	34
7. aspirin	32
8. insulin	16
9. dextropropoxyphene	16
10. chlormethiazole	13

Fig. 8.1 The top ten agents responsible for fatal self-poisoning. This does not necessarily correlate with the relative numbers presenting with an overdose of the corresponding medication (e.g. benzodiazepine overdose is common, but rarely fatal). (OPCS, Office of Population Censuses and Surveys mortality statistics)

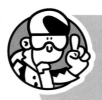

Remember that the history is often unreliable, especially on presentation, for a variety of reasons.

Establish the time between taking the medication and presentation

There may be little benefit in performing gastric lavage or forced emesis more than four hours after the overdose unless the drug delays gastric emptying (e.g. tricyclic antidepressants). If there is any uncertainty, it is probably better to perform a gastric lavage.

Explore the circumstances of the action

This will help to assess suicidal intention. Certain characteristics are more typical of those patients who take a fatal overdose than those who do not (Fig. 8.2).

Review the events surrounding the episode directly, for example:
- Was the patient alone at the time?
- Were special measures taken to avoid or ensure discovery?
- Was a suicide note written?
- Had anyone else been warned about the attempt either before or after?
- Ask: "Did you intend to kill yourself?"
- Ask: "Are you pleased that you are still alive?"
- Did the patient think that the agent taken in the dose used was potentially fatal?

Review recent life events that may have acted as a precipitant for the overdose. Explore the events that directly led up to the ingestion of medication (e.g. bereavement, termination of a relationship, marital difficulties, stress at work, financial problems).

Past medical history

A detailed psychiatric history is essential. Concentrate on previous attempts at deliberate self-harm (e.g. drug overdose, self-mutilation) and specifically consider other

63

Characteristics of patients more likely to take a deliberately fatal or non-fatal drug overdose		
Characteristic	Fatal overdose	Non-fatal overdose
age group	older	adolescent, young adult
male versus female	male > female	female > male
social background	socially isolated, unemployed	lives with family/friends
health	pre-existing psychiatric or medical (especially chronic) disorder	previously well or personality disorder
drug/alcohol abuse	drug and alcohol abuse	less likely

Fig. 8.2 Background characteristics of patients more likely to take a fatal or non-fatal drug overdose deliberately.

psychiatric illnesses (e.g. depression). Review past medical history. In particular, consider chronic painful or terminal illnesses.

Drug history

Review current medication, especially psychotropic drugs. Ask specifically about use of drugs of abuse and alcohol. Consider how the patient gained access to the medication consumed (e.g. own supply, from a shop, used mother's 'tranquillizers').

Family history

Enquire about any family history of self-poisoning or psychiatric illness. If other family members have taken drug overdoses, what did they take, and what was the end result?

Social history

A detailed social history often puts the event in perspective. Concentrate on the immediate family and home environment. Consider sources of conflict and stress, as well as support.

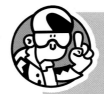

Patients seen on first contact after an episode of deliberate self-harm are often reluctant historians. Obtain the basic information needed to institute emergency care, but this is no substitute for a full history at a later stage.

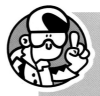

Attempt to elicit information on three components:
- **Mechanics of the overdose (medication, dose, time).**
- **Immediate precipitating events.**
- **Background family and interpersonal relationships and stresses in life.**

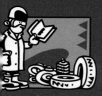

9. Presenting Problems: Locomotor System

Detailed history

Back pain is extremely common. The history is used to highlight potentially serious or treatable causes of the pain. Consider the differential diagnosis of back pain (Fig. 9.1).

Ask patients what they consider to be the cause of the pain. This is always extremely informative. Take a detailed history in the usual systematic manner, focusing on the factors below.

Location of the pain

Most back pain is in the lumbar region. Thoracic pain is usually due to an organic cause (e.g. tuberculosis, osteoporotic crush fracture, myeloma).

Radiation of the pain

For example, radiation down the distribution of the sciatic nerve after lumbar disc prolapse.

Speed of onset

This may be acute (e.g. disc prolapse, crush fracture), subacute (e.g. malignancy, infection, inflammatory causes), or chronic for years (non-specific back pain, psychogenic).

Aggravating and relieving factors

Mechanical pain is often exacerbated by exercise. Inflammatory pain is often worse after a period of inactivity. Spinal stenosis may be worse on walking, but relieved by leaning forwards or resting.

Pattern of severity with time

For example, is the patient experiencing chronic unrelenting pain (e.g. inflammatory disease, psychogenic), intermittent or relapsing pain (e.g. disc disease).

Associated symptoms

A full review of systems enquiry should be performed as

Differential diagnosis of back pain

inflammatory
  ankylosing spondylitis*; psoriatic arthropathy; enteropathic arthropathy; Whipple's disease

bone disease
  osteoporosis*; osteomalacia; renal bone disease; malignancy

disc disease and osteoarthritis
  spondylosis*, acute disc prolapse*; tuberculosis and septic discitis

mechanical disease
  posture* (pregnancy, obesity, scoliosis, etc.); spondylolisthesis; spinal stenosis

soft tissue disease
  'fibrositis'*; muscle strain*

psychogenic
  make a positive diagnosis (somatisation, chronic backpain with psychological or social sequelae

non-specific back pain*
  the most common cause; usually has a mechanical basis

referred pain
  chronic pancreatitis; posterior duodenal ulcer; abdominal aortic aneurysm, etc.

Fig. 9.1 Differential diagnosis of back pain. * indicates the more common causes.

the back pain may be part of a systemic disease such as ankylosing spondylosis (polyarthritis, dyspnoea), malignancy, renal failure.

Medical history

A detailed medical history may elicit a potential underlying cause for the pain. Consider psychiatric disorders, especially depression, which may be a cause or result of the pain.

Drug history

Ask patients what analgesics they have taken in an attempt to relieve the symptoms and their efficacy.

Social history

Explore how the pain limits functional activity. Ask specifically about time off work due to the pain. For suspected non-specific pain or psychogenic pain, explore current social pressures being experienced by the patient.

Review of systems enquiry

It is essential to consider systemic illnesses that may have precipitated the pain. In particular, consider weight loss, fevers, sweats, features suggestive of malignancy, and polyarthritis

Back pain is very common. A good history is the key to efficient diagnosis and can prevent unnecessary and occasionally expensive or unpleasant investigations, which may reinforce illness behaviour.

Try to distinguish between systemic disease and mechanical pain. Symptoms such as thoracic pain, weight loss, fevers, systemic symptoms, or new-onset pain should trigger further investigation for organic pathology.

Psychogenic back pain is not a diagnosis of exclusion. An attempt to make a positive diagnosis should be made as management can be tailored to this.

RHEUMATOID ARTHRITIS

Detailed history

Rheumatoid arthritis is a multisystem disease and the history should be taken in a systematic manner.

Background disease

Ask about age of onset (typically 25–40 years) and usual pattern of arthritis.

Current disease activity

Attempt to assess whether the patient has active synovitis and try to distinguish it from secondary osteoarthritis due to burnt out rheumatoid disease. Enquire about the time pattern of disease activity (e.g. relentless progression, disease flares separated by periods of remission) and the presence of red or swollen joints. Note the response to analgesics and non-steroidal anti-inflammatory drugs (NSAIDs) and the duration of early morning stiffness (> 30 minutes is significant). Map out the joints that the patient thinks are inflamed (Fig. 9.2).

Functional impact of the disease

Consider how current disease activity has altered functional ability. For example, ask: "Is there anything that you have difficulty doing now that you could manage a few weeks ago?". Consider mobility and grip. Ascertain whether activities are limited by pain, weakness, or other factors.

Extra-articular features of the disease

Rheumatoid arthritis should be considered as a systemic disease. For each system, consider how disease activity may be manifested:

- Lung—dyspnoea (e.g. due to rheumatoid nodules, pleural effusion, bronchiolitis obliterans).

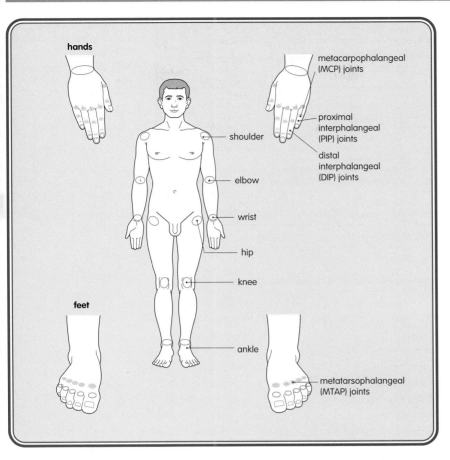

Fig. 9.2 Simple diagrams can be used to illustrate the distribution of active synovitis. Shaded circles represent inflamed joints. Open circles indicate non-inflamed joints.

Labels in figure:
hands
metacarpophalangeal (MCP) joints
shoulder
proximal interphalangeal (PIP) joints
distal interphalangeal (DIP) joints
elbow
wrist
hip
knee
feet
ankle
metatarsophalangeal (MTAP) joints

- Skin—rash, vasculitic leg ulcers, rheumatoid nodules.
- Nervous system—paraesthesiae (especially carpal tunnel syndrome), symptoms of peripheral neuropathy.
- Eyes—dry eyes (Sjögren's syndrome) especially if associated with a dry mouth, red eye (scleritis).
- Renal—proteinuria or known dysfunction (e.g. due to amyloid, medication).

Drug history

A particularly detailed drug history is absolutely essential. Concentrate on drugs currently being used to control the disease (e.g. glucocorticosteroids, analgesics, NSAIDs, second-line agents). Often, a multitude of drug combinations has been used previously. Try to chart previous experiences objectively so that an assessment can be made about changing agents, if necessary, to improve control of disease activity. For each second-line drug, chart the:

- Duration of use.
- Efficacy—use objective parameters if possible, for example erythrocyte sedimentation rate (ESR), early morning stiffness, progression of joint erosions radiologically.
- Reason for discontinuation—for example side effects, lack of response.
- Doses used—especially cumulative dose.

All second-line agents have side effects (Fig. 9.3). Ask specifically about the use of glucocorticosteroids.

Social history

It is important to investigate the functional impact of the disease on daily life, exploring the home environment as well as occupation. Many aids to living are available, and specialist use of physiotherapists and occupational therapists may be invaluable.

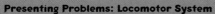

Side effects of second-line agents used in the treatment of rheumatoid arthritis	
Drug	**Side effects**
gold	proteinuria (membranous nephropathy); thrombocytopenia and agranulocytosis; skin rash (approximately 25%); stomatitis
penicillamine	proteinuria (common); nephrotic syndrome; thrombocytopenia; agranulocytosis; anorexia; nausea (early in treatment); rash
methotrexate	bone marrow suppression; oral ulceration; gastrointestinal disturbances; hepatotoxicity (especially prolonged use); teratogenic
azathioprine	bone marrow suppression; increased risk of malignancy; infections; gastrointestinal disturbances
sulphasalazine	nausea; vomiting; skin rash; blood dyscrasia (rare)
hydroxychloroquine	retinopathy (especially long-term use)

Fig. 9.3 Side effects of second-line agents used in the treatment of rheumatoid arthritis.

Remember that rheumatoid arthritis is a chronic (and often disabling) condition. Patient education and motivation are crucial for optimal rehabilitation. It is particularly important that a feeling of mutual trust is fostered between the patient and doctor.

10. Presenting Problems: Endocrine System

THE DIABETIC PATIENT

Detailed history
Review presentation with diabetes mellitus
The most important features are:
- Age of onset.
- Presenting symptoms (e.g. weight loss, polyuria, polydipsia, coma).

Form of diabetes mellitus
Note the class of disease, as complications and management stategies will vary, for example:
- Type I—insulin-dependent diabetes mellitus (IDDM).
- Type II—non-insulin-dependent diabetes mellitus (NIDDM) or insulin-requiring diabetes mellitus.
- Secondary (due to glucocorticosteroids, pancreatitis, Cushing's disease).

Diabetic control
This is the cornerstone of managing diabetes mellitus, so much of the time available at consultation should be devoted to this. Review the form of blood sugar control (e.g. diet alone, oral hypoglycaemic agents, insulin).

Establish how the patient monitors glycaemic control. Check the form of monitoring (e.g. measuring blood glucose, urinalysis), frequency of measurements, and the levels attained. Most patients will have a book charting the blood glucose level. This should be reviewed to assess general control and fluctuations at different times of the day. It also provides an insight into the patient's concordance. In an analogous way to checking inhaler technique (see p. 28), it is often informative to observe a patient performing a blood glucose estimate.

Complications
Complications of diabetic control
Review the frequency of acute complications of therapy or hyperglycaemia, for example:
- Hypoglycaemic attacks.
- Hyperosmolar non-ketotic coma.
- Diabetic ketoacidosis (DKA).

Ask specifically about symptoms suggestive of poor control, for example:
- Weight loss, malaise, fatigue.
- Polyuria, polydipsia (due to osmotic diuresis).
- Blurred vision (refractive changes in the eye).
- Balanitis, pruritus vulvae, thrush.

Macrovascular complications
Diabetes mellitus is strongly associated with macrovascular disease. It is imperative that any coincident risk factors are eliminated. Check for symptoms related to the three main forms of macrovascular disease:
- Ischaemic heart disease (ask specifically about chest pains, myocardial infarction).
- Peripheral vascular disease (e.g. claudication).
- Cerebrovascular disease.

Microvascular complications
Long-term disease is associated with relentless progression of microvascular disease. Early recognition may allow specific therapy to be instituted. Ask about the three main forms of microvascular disease:
- Retinopathy—ask about visual symptoms, laser therapy.
- Neuropathy—paraesthesiae.
- Nephropathy—proteinuria and hypertension.

Other complications
Diabetes mellitus is associated with other complications, which may be multifactorial. Specific enquiry should be made about:
- Impotence—rarely spontaneously volunteered by the patient, but common.
- Staphylococcal skin infections—for example boils, carbuncles.
- Gastroparesis—nausea, vomiting, early satiety.
- Foot ulcers—neuropathy and vasculopathy.

Past medical history
Review the other risk factors for ischaemic heart and cerebrovascular disease. Consider other possible

autoimmune diseases (especially thyroiditis, pernicious anaemia, vitiligo, Addison's disease), renal failure, and systemic infections.

Drug history
Review the agents used to control the diabetes.

Oral hypoglycaemic agents
Consider whether it is appropriate for the patient to be on an oral hypoglycaemic agent. Beware of metformin in the presence of renal dysfunction (metformin is contra-indicated as it may cause lactic acidosis). Consider whether it is more appropriate to use agents that are hepatically metabolized or renally excreted.

Insulin
Review the form of insulin used (e.g. long or short acting, porcine or human). Assess whether the dose needs to be modified. Ask about problems at injection sites (e.g. lipohypertrophy, scarring).

Review the use of other medication that may aggravate diabetic control (e.g. glucocorticosteroids, thiazide diuretics). It may be possible to improve diabetic control by appropriate adjustment of other medication.

Family history
This is usually positive for type II diabetes mellitus.

Social history
Review home circumstances, for example:
- Is the patient's eyesight good enough to read blood glucose sticks?
- Does the patient have sufficient manual dexterity (especially if he or she had neuropathy) to monitor his or her own therapy?

Education and motivation are central to the long-term outlook for the diabetic patient. An appropriate diet is essential for improving the control of all diabetic patients, especially those who are obese. Help from a dietician may be indicated. It is particularly important that the patient understands the unacceptable risks of smoking.

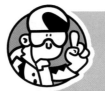

In diabetes mellitus, patient education and motivation are crucial to the long-term prognosis. Good long-term control is pivotal for reducing the long-term complications of diabetes mellitus. Focus on risk factors for ischaemic heart disease and always ask specifically about visual problems and foot care.

THYROID DISEASE

Presenting complaint
Hypothyroidism and hyperthyroidism may present in many ways, and form part of the differential diagnosis of a variety of disorders. Some of the more common presentations are shown in Fig. 10.1. A high index of suspicion may be needed to diagnose these conditions as presentation is often non-specific.

Detailed history
Hyperthyroidism
Ask about symptoms of hyperthyroidism. Enquire specifically about palpitations.

The common causes of atrial fibrillation are ischaemic heart disease, hyperthyroidism, and mitral valve disease.

The following specific features may suggest underlying Graves' disease:
- Eye disease (diplopia, proptosis).
- Goitre.
- Pretibial myxoedema.

Hypothyroidism

Ask about symptoms of hypothyroidism (see Fig. 10.1). In particular, enquire about weight gain, fertility problems, menstrual difficulties, and cold intolerance. The symptoms are often insidious and are not noticed by patients or their immediate family, but may be observed by occasional visitors or general practitioners.

Past medical history

Ask about:

- Other autoimmune disorders (e.g. diabetes mellitus, Addison's disease, vitiligo, myasthenia gravis).

- Previous partial thyroidectomy or treatment with radio-iodine if there is suspected hypothyroidism.

Also consider secondary treatable causes of thyroid disease (Fig. 10.2) and the presence of ischaemic heart disease in hypothyroid patients as therapy will then need to be more cautious.

Drug history

Review the use and dose of antithyroid medication and thyroxine. Consider drugs that may aggravate symptoms (e.g. β-blockers causing bradycardia in

Presenting features of thyroid disease	
Hypothyroidism	**Hyperthyroidism**
weight gain*	weight loss despite good appetite*
general slowness	
mental slowing, poor memory	poor concentration
anorexia	
cold intolerance*	heat intolerance*, excessive sweating
depression	agitation*, restlessness*
coma	
constipation	diarrhoea
altered appearance	eye changes
	palpitations

Fig. 10.1 Presenting features of thyroid disease. * indicates more common or discriminatory features.

Secondary causes of thyroid disease	
Hypothyroidism	**Hyperthyroidism**
dietary iodine deficiency	
antithyroid drugs used at inappropriate dose or on resolution of hyperthyroid state	over-dosage with thyroxine
post-thyroid surgery	
radio-iodine therapy	thyroid carcinoma (rare)
tumour infiltration (rare)	TSH-secreting tumours (rare)
hypopituitarism	acute thyroiditis (e.g. infective, autoimmune)
post-subacute thyroiditis	

Fig. 10.2 Secondary causes of thyroid disease. (TSH, thyroid-stimulating hormone.)

hypothyroidism). In addition, consider drugs that may interfere with interpretation of thyroid function tests (e.g. oestrogens increase thyroid-binding globulin concentration). Thyroid-stimulating hormone (TSH) levels are often needed in addition to total thyroxine concentration, when interpreting thyroid function tests.

Review of systems enquiry

A detailed screen of systemic symptoms is essential as many features are non-specific. It is often fruitful to concentrate on mental changes.

 Try to assess thyroid status clinically in treated patients as biochemical tests lag behind therapeutic responses by several weeks.

 **Hypothyroidism and hyperthyroidism can produce a multitude of symptoms. A high index of suspicion is needed, particularly in the context of mental changes, palpitations, changes in weight, altered conscious level, or cardiac disease. The most discriminatory features from the history are cold and heat intolerance and weight changes despite contradictory dietary history. A relative may provide invaluable clues as the patient may not spontaneously report symptoms.**

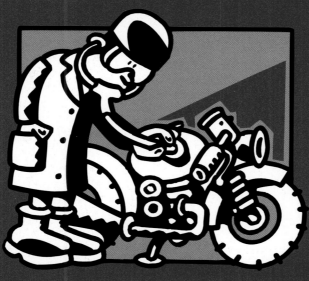

EXAMINATION

11. Introduction

SETTING

A good physical examination relies upon a cooperative patient and a well-lit room. It is important to engender an atmosphere of trust and professionalism during the history taking and to explain the steps of the examination appropriately, and if necessary what information you hope to elicit from the process. This will help to avoid any misunderstanding and will reassure the patient, taking away some of the mysticism that may surround the doctor–patient relationship. For example, many patients are surprised when a doctor starts an examination of the abdomen by becoming engrossed in their nails! It is important to be sensitive to the patient. Consider whether it is appropriate for a chaperone to be present or, conversely, whether it is inappropriate for the patient's partner to be in the room during the examination.

The patient must be appropriately positioned, comfortable, and in a well-lit warm room. Ensure that there is adequate privacy. It is clearly unacceptable for a semi-clad patient to be examined on a couch without screens if the door to the examination room is potentially going to be opened without warning!

EXAMINATION ROUTINE

Although the examination is described as a separate process from the history, a good assessment should start as soon as the patient walks into the examination room (Fig. 11.1). There are countless other observations that can be made, and a rapid inspection of the patient will put the subsequently elicited history into context.

The examination, like the history, should be performed in a systematic manner, but again it is vital to be aware of the differential diagnosis as each sign is elicited. Once again the process is active. The examination routine usually follows a strict order. For most systems, the order of examination is as follows:

- Inspection.
- Palpation.
- Percussion.
- Auscultation.

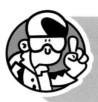

The most important component of the examination is inspection.

EXAMINING A SYSTEM

When examining any system, try to answer the following three questions.

What is the pathology?

This process requires interpretation of the physical signs so that a deviation from normality can be recognized and the individual signs integrated.

What is the aetiology of the pathological process?

It is not enough to identify that a patient has a pleural effusion. An attempt should be made to find the underlying cause (e.g. lymphadenopathy and

---

Points to consider when the patient walks into the room

Does the patient look ill or in pain?

Is the patient cachectic or overweight?

What is the patient's racial origin?

Does the patient have a normal gait?

Is the patient short of breath on walking into the examination room?

Does the patient require help to get out of a chair?

Fig. 11.1 Points to consider when the patient walks into the room.

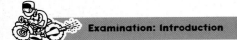

hepatomegaly suggesting malignancy, a third heart sound and elevated jugular venous pressure suggesting heart failure and fluid overload).

What is the severity and functional impact on the patient?

For example, severe aortic stenosis is an indication for valve replacement. This may be assessed clinically by measuring the pulse pressure and noting the presence of a slow-rising pulse.

PHYSICAL SIGNS

Many physical signs are subtle, or simply represent a qualitative change from normal. It is essential that the doctor has an appreciation of the wide range of normality so that any signs can be placed into context. There are no short cuts. To gain this ability requires practice.

OVERVIEW OF EXAMINATION SECTION

This section of the book is divided into the individual systems of the body. The first part of each chapter describes the routine examination of that system. The second part illustrates the process described above in practice by providing examples of pathologies or presentations related to the system. These examples are intended to provide a skeleton for the student's examination, illustrating the important features. Remember that the examination is a highly individual skill, and with experience students should adopt their own style within the framework of the general examination. It is important to get as much feedback as possible on your examination technique. Take every opportunity for someone more experienced to be present, to watch what you are doing, and give you constructive feedback.

The cardiovascular examination is particularly satisfying as the physical signs elicited can usually be correlated with the pathophysiology. Many cardiovascular pathologies produce multiple signs which, when integrated, allow assessment of the severity and aetiology of the lesion. It is particularly important to perform the examination in a systematic manner so that physical signs can be put into context with each other.

Patient exposure and position
Ensure adequate lighting. The patient should be comfortable and seated at 45 degrees to the horizontal, and stripped to the waist. Female patients should remove their bra. (It is difficult auscultating through clothing!) It is courteous to provide a blanket as the patient may wish to remain covered until examination of the precordium.

General inspection
In all systems, the specific examination should be preceded by an inspection of the patient. Vital clues are often found.

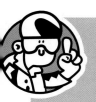

It is essential to know in advance what you are looking for, or it will not be found! Prepare a mental checklist. The whole process need take only a few seconds.

General features
Note any obvious features on general observation, including:
- Age, sex, general health.
- Body habitus (obese or cachectic).
- Dyspnoea (observe the effort required to climb onto the couch).

Listen for any clicks of prosthetic heart valves. Inspection can then be performed from the head downwards.

Eyes
A brief inspection will reveal abnormalities such as arcus senilis (significant in young adults, suggesting hypercholesterolaemia) or xanthelasma (suggestive of hyperlipidaemia). The patient may be obviously jaundiced.

Face
Look for evidence of cyanosis (requires at least 5 g/dL deoxygenated haemoglobin), particularly around the lips or under the tongue, or plethora (e.g. due to superior vena cava obstruction (SVCO), polycythaemia). The patient may have a facies typical of a pathological process, for example:
- Malar flush (mitral stenosis).
- 'Elfin' facies (congenital aortic stenosis).

Always inspect the mouth (poor dental hygiene may be the cause of infective endocarditis).

Neck
Note any visible pulsations (e.g. due to tricuspid regurgitation, aortic regurgitation).

Precordium
Observe the shape of the chest for:
- Any obvious deformity (e.g. pectus excavatum in Marfan's syndrome).
- Visible collateral veins (e.g. in superior vena cava obstruction).
- Visible apex beat (e.g. left ventricular hypertrophy).
- Presence of any scars (Fig. 12.1).

Also look in the brachial and femoral regions for scars from cardiac catheterization.

Ankles
Briefly look for swelling suggestive of peripheral oedema. This can be confirmed by later examination.

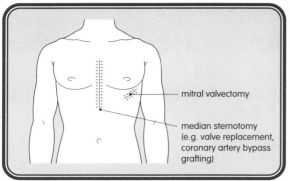

mitral valvectomy

median sternotomy
(e.g. valve replacement,
coronary artery bypass
grafting)

Fig. 12.1 Position of scars related to cardiovascular pathology on the praecordium.

Specific examination

Specific examination can now be performed.

Hands

Careful examination of the hands often reveals clues of underlying cardiovascular disease. Feel the temperature and look for peripheral cyanosis. Note the shape of the hands (e.g. arachnodactyly in Marfan's syndrome).

Clubbing

The cardinal feature of clubbing is loss of angle of the nailfold. Other features include increased convex curvature in both a longitudinal and transverse plane,

Adequate inspection is neglected at your peril! If omitted, simple diagnoses can be easily overlooked. It also helps to anticipate subsequently elicited physical signs and to put them in perspective.

increased fluctuation of the nailbed, and swelling of the terminal phalanx (Fig. 12.2). Remember to look at both hands. Clubbing can rarely be detected in the toes. Hold the nail up to the plane of your eyes to facilitate detection. Although a non-specific sign, its presence should alert the physician to underlying disease (Fig. 12.3).

New-onset clubbing is highly significant. If detected, ask the patient whether he or she has noticed any recent change in the shape of their nails.

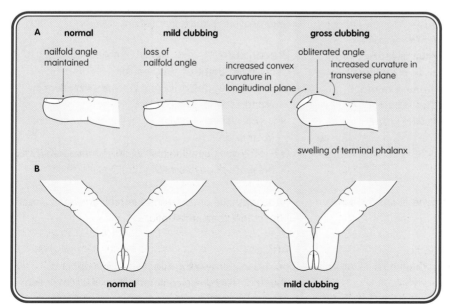

Fig. 12.2 (A) Features of clubbing. The cardinal sign is loss of angle of the nailfold. (B) If the patient is asked to place his index fingers 'back to back', the diamond-shaped gap normally present is obliterated in early clubbing.

Causes of clubbing	
System	**Disease associations**
cardiovascular	infective endocarditis* (late sign); congenital cyanotic heart disease; atrial myxoma (very rare)
respiratory	carcinoma of the bronchus*; fibrosing alveolitis*; chronic suppurative lung disease* (empyema, bronchiectasis, pulmonary abscess, cystic fibrosis)
abdominal	Crohn's disease (unusual); cirrhosis
familial	most common cause*

Fig. 12.3 Causes of clubbing. * indicates the more common causes.

Splinter haemorrhages

Splinter haemorrhages (Fig. 12.4) are a feature of a vasculitic process (see infective endocarditis, p. 94), but the most common cause is mild trauma, and a small number (e.g. < 5) is normal.

Nailfold infarcts

Nailfold infarcts (Fig. 12.4) are also a feature of vasculitis, but more specific than splinter haemorrhages. They are often associated with other features of infective endocarditis (see infective endocarditis, p. 94).

Capillary return

Apart from noting the temperature of the skin, peripheral perfusion may be assessed by capillary return. Light digital pressure to the end of the nail will produce blanching. The speed of capillary return can be visualized. Poor peripheral perfusion can be easily detected. Visible pulsation may be seen in aortic regurgitation.

Nicotine staining

Cigarette staining of the fingertips and nails may counter information given in the history.

Other signs of infective endocarditis

Look for other rare stigmata of infective endocarditis, for example:

- Osler's nodes (tender nodules on the finger pulps).
- Janeway lesions (see infective endocarditis, p. 94).

Xanthomas

Lipid deposition may occur in tendons, skin, or soft tissues in some hyperlipidaemic states, for example:

- Tendon xanthomas (especially of Achilles tendon,

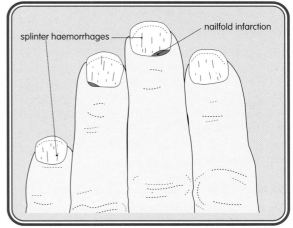

Fig. 12.4 Splinter haemorrhages and nailfold infarcts. If both lesions appear together, infective endocarditis or a vasculitic process is highly likely.

extensor tendons on hands)—type II hyperlipidaemia.
- Palmar xanthomas (skin creases of palms and soles)— type III hyperlipidaemia.

Arterial pulse

The arterial pulse may be palpated at various sites (Fig. 12.5). The pulse has various characteristics, which should be defined in each patient.

Presence and symmetry

Compare the radial pulsations synchronously (asymmetry may be detectable in certain conditions such as large vessel vasculitis, Takayasu's, aortic dissection). Obstruction may delay the pulse. Check for radiofemoral delay, especially in hypertension (e.g. due to coarctation of the

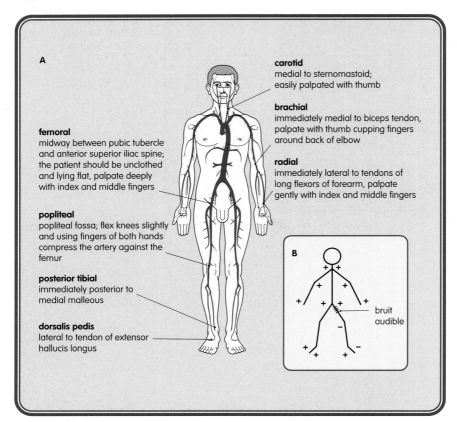

Fig. 12.5 (A) Location of the arterial pulses. (B) Typical notation in the hospital records. (+, pulse present; –, pulse not palpable).

A

carotid
medial to sternomastoid; easily palpated with thumb

brachial
immediately medial to biceps tendon, palpate with thumb cupping fingers around back of elbow

radial
immediately lateral to tendons of long flexors of forearm, palpate gently with index and middle fingers

femoral
midway between pubic tubercle and anterior superior iliac spine; the patient should be unclothed and lying flat, palpate deeply with index and middle fingers

popliteal
popliteal fossa; flex knees slightly and using fingers of both hands compress the artery against the femur

posterior tibial
immediately posterior to medial malleous

dorsalis pedis
lateral to tendon of extensor hallucis longus

B

bruit audible

aorta). Assess the presence of each pulse, especially if there is embolism or peripheral artery disease.

Rate
Normal pulse rate is 60–100/minute. Count for at least 15 seconds at the radial pulse. This may also provide an opportunity for additional visual inspection of the patient. The radial pulse rate may differ from the number of ventricular contractions per minute (e.g. apicoradial deficit in fast atrial fibrillation). Consider the rate within the clinical context (e.g. tachycardia in the presence of fever, hypovolaemia; bradycardia in hypothermia, hypothyroidism).

Rhythm
The normal pulse rhythm is regular sinus rhythm. Any irregularity should be characterized, and if possible confirmed by an electrocardiogram (ECG). Many arrhythmias are characteristic (Fig. 12.6). Try to establish whether the underlying rhythm is regular (e.g. frequent ectopic beats) or chaotic (e.g. atrial fibrillation).

Volume
Pulse volume reflects stroke volume. This is best assessed at the carotid or brachial pulse. There is a wide range of 'normal'. It is important to practise on as many different patients as possible so that you can recognize when abnormal signs are present.
  Some of the abnormalities of pulse volume include:
- Pulsus paradoxus. This is detectable in cardiac tamponade or severe asthma. The pulse becomes weak or absent on inpiration. Pulsus paradoxus reflects an exaggeration of the normal physiological changes in intrathoracic pressure and the influence of the diaphragm and interventricular septal changes during the respiratory cycle.
- Pulsus alternans. This is a sign of severe left ventricular failure. Alternate pulses are felt as strong or weak due to the presence of bigeminy.
- Coarctation of the aorta. As well as radiofemoral delay (described above), the pulse volume of the femoral pulse is usually noticeably reduced.

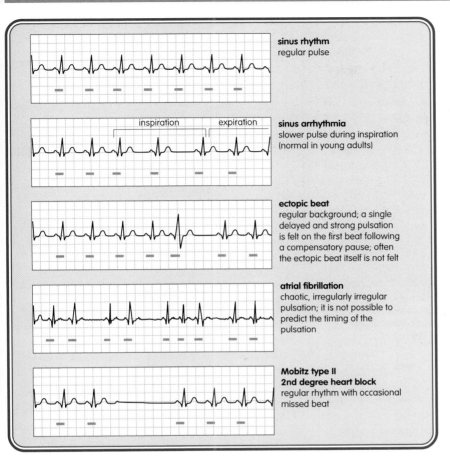

Fig. 12.6 Common arrhythmias. In each recording the upper trace is the ECG and the lower trace illustrates a bar corresponding to each palpable pulsation. It is often possible to elucidate the underlying rhythm disturbance.

Within the figure:

sinus rhythm
regular pulse

inspiration   expiration

sinus arrhythmia
slower pulse during inspiration (normal in young adults)

ectopic beat
regular background; a single delayed and strong pulsation is felt on the first beat following a compensatory pause; often the ectopic beat itself is not felt

atrial fibrillation
chaotic, irregularly irregular pulsation; it is not possible to predict the timing of the pulsation

Mobitz type II
2nd degree heart block
regular rhythm with occasional missed beat

Character

With increasing distance from the aorta, particularly in sclerotic vessels, the waveform becomes distorted (Fig. 12.7), so volume and character should be assessed using either the carotid or brachial pulses. A picture of the waveform often correlates with the severity of valvular disorders. This sign requires considerable practice to elicit, so that the range of normality can be appreciated. It is only by knowing the normal range that abnormalities in pulse character can be recognised. Try to become used to the pulse character of the common pathologies (Fig. 12.8).

Blood pressure

As with other components of the cardiovascular examination, it is important to adopt a systematic approach, for example as follows:

- Allow the patient to relax—white coat hypertension is a real phenomenon.

- Make sure the cuff is placed centrally over the brachial artery.
- Use a large cuff in obese subjects with an arm circumference over 30 cm (a common cause of overestimating blood pressure is to use a too small cuff).
- On deflating the cuff, note the point of the first audible sounds (Korotkov I), the point at which sounds become muffled (Korotkov IV), and the point of disappearance of sounds (Korotkov V, which is usually 5–10 mm Hg lower than phase IV, but occasionally 0 mm Hg. Use phase V as a record of diastolic pressure as this produces less interobserver error.

Occasionally, additional blood pressure readings are indicated:
- Postural—for example if the patient is on

Cardiovascular Examination

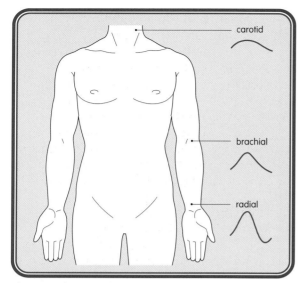

Fig. 12.7 Changing character of the pulse waveform with distance from the heart. This is particularly marked in sclerotic vessels. Even in severe aortic stenosis the waveform may appear normal at the radial pulse.

Description	Waveform	Associations
normal		—
slow rising		aortic stenosis
collapsing (water hammer)		aortic regurgitation persistent ductus arteriosus

Fig. 12.8 Typical arterial waveforms palpated at the carotid pulse in different conditions. The waveform often provides important information about the severity of the underlying pathology.

antihypertensive medication or has dizziness, or to assess hypovolaemia.
- Comparison of right and left arms—for example for aortic dissection, aortic coarctation.
- Repeated measurements—before diagnosing hypertension, always take readings on a variety of occasions.
- Pulsus paradoxus —for example for asthma, cardiac tamponade.
- Comparison of the ankle:brachial ratio—for example for aortic coarctation, peripheral vascular disease.

The blood pressure is a vital sign, so should be elicited with great care and given the respect that it deserves! It should be measured to the nearest 2 mm Hg.

Neck
Arterial pulse
Follow the usual pattern of:
- Inspection—look at the pulsation (e.g. signs of collapsing pulse—Corrigan's sign, de Musset's

sign—see aortic regurgitation, p. 90).
- Palpation—palpate the carotid artery specifically for volume and character.
- Auscultation—auscultate for the presence of a carotid bruit.

Venous pulse
Assessment of the jugular venous waveform is of fundamental importance to the cardiovascular examination (Fig. 12.9). There are no valves between the right atrium and internal jugular vein, which is readily distensible. Therefore it can act as a manometer reflecting the filling pressure of the right heart. Examine the height of the wave. The jugular venous pressure (JVP) is measured as the vertical height of the column of blood in the internal jugular vein above the sternal angle (Fig. 12.10).

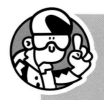
Assessment of the JVP should not be neglected. It is the most direct assessment of the filling pressure of the right heart.

The venous pulsation should be distinguished from arterial pulsation (Fig. 12.11). If it is not visible, the pressure may be:

- Too low (e.g. in hypovolaemia)—lie the patient flat, test the hepatojugular reflux.

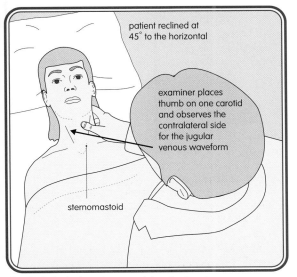

patient reclined at 45° to the horizontal

examiner places thumb on one carotid and observes the contralateral side for the jugular venous waveform

sternomastoid

Fig. 12.9 Technique for examining the jugular venous waveform. Place a thumb over the carotid artery to time any pulsations and observe the deflections on the contralateral side produced by the pressure waveform in the internal jugular vein. The waveform is usually just visible above the clavicle.

- Too high (e.g. in right ventricular infarction, volume overload)—sit the patient upright.

Note the character of the waveform. A basic appreciation of the normal jugular venous waveform is needed (Fig. 12.12). Assessment of the waveform requires considerable skill and experience. Unfortunately there are no short cuts. Assessment may give clues to pathologies such as tricuspid regurgitation (giant v waves), atrial fibrillation (no atrial systole, so only one component), complete heart block (cannon waves).

Precordium

Although this is the meat of the cardiovascular examination, clues to underlying pathology should have been derived from the peripheral examination. Follow a strict examination routine. Remember that palpation should precede auscultation.

Apex beat

The apex beat is the most downward and outward position where the cardiac impulse is palpable. Define the following.

Position: The normal apex beat is within the fifth intercostal space in the midclavicular line (Fig. 12.13). A displaced apex beat usually implies volume overload of the left ventricle.

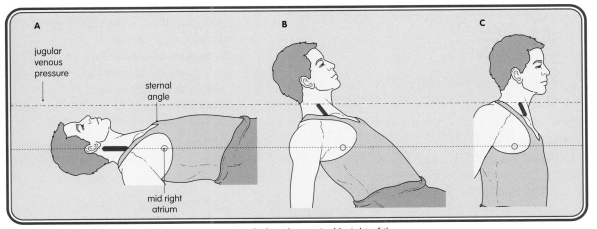

A

jugular venous pressure

sternal angle

mid right atrium

B

C

Fig. 12.10 The jugular venous pressure (JVP) is recorded as the vertical height of the visible waveform above the sternal angle. The pressure is fixed, but the anatomical position of the waveform varies according to posture. The jugular venous pressure is usually 2–5 cm H_2O. The dark line corresponds to the distended jugular vein visible above the clavicle. As the patient alters his or her posture, the amount of visibly distended vein alters as the vertical height is fixed.

Characteristics of the jugular venous waveform and arterial pulse in the neck	
Jugular venous pulse	**Carotid pulse**
most prominent deflection is inwards	most prominent deflection is outwards
in sinus rhythm, two deflections for each beat	only one deflection for each beat
height of the wave changes with posture	height is independent of posture
temporary elevation of wave following pressure over the right costal margin (hepatojugular reflux)	constant
can usually be eliminated by light digital pressure over the clavicles	still present after light pressure
not palpable (in absence of tricuspid regurgitation)	palpable

Fig. 12.11 Characteristics of the jugular venous waveform and arterial pulse in the neck.

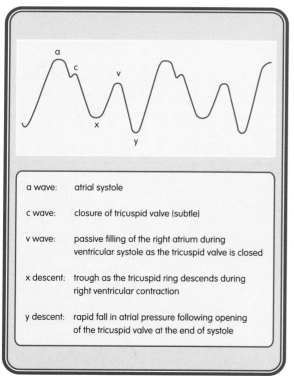

a wave:	atrial systole
c wave:	closure of tricuspid valve (subtle)
v wave:	passive filling of the right atrium during ventricular systole as the tricuspid valve is closed
x descent:	trough as the tricuspid ring descends during right ventricular contraction
y descent:	rapid fall in atrial pressure following opening of the tricuspid valve at the end of systole

Fig. 12.12 The components of the jugular venous waveform. In practice, the c wave is not usually visible. It is only by understanding the normal waveform that pathognomonic signs such as cannon waves and giant v waves can be recognized.

 Pressure overload (e.g. in aortic stenosis, hypertension) causes left ventricular hypertrophy. The left ventricle hypertrophies from the outside inwards so, unless there is also cardiac failure, it should not displace the apex beat. Volume overload (e.g. in aortic regurgitation) causes left ventricular dilatation and consequent displacement of the apex beat.

Character: Check the character of the beat. For example:
- Forceful, 'sustained', 'heaving'—left ventricular hypertrophy.
- Tapping—mitral stenosis.
- Thrusting—volume overload.

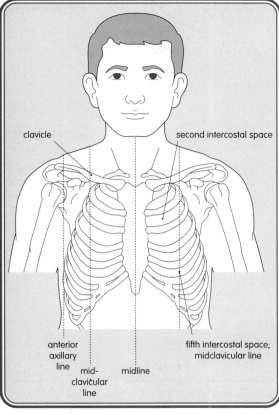

Fig. 12.13 Surface anatomy of the apex beat. It is defined in relation to the intercostal space and imaginary vertical lines related to the clavicle and axilla. The normal apex beat is within the fifth intercostal space in the midclavicular line.

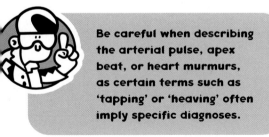

Be careful when describing the arterial pulse, apex beat, or heart murmurs, as certain terms such as 'tapping' or 'heaving' often imply specific diagnoses.

Palpating the rest of the precordium

Note the presence of:

- Heaves—use either the palm or the medial aspect of the hand; right ventricular hypertrophy may cause a left parasternal lifting sensation.
- Thrills—palpable murmurs (especially in aortic stenosis) feel like a fly trapped in one's hands.

- Palpable heart sounds—for example first heart sound in mitral stenosis.

Auscultation

An understanding of the cardiac cycle is essential when interpreting findings (Fig. 12.14). When auscultating, place your thumb on the carotid so that heart sounds and murmurs can be timed in relation to systole (Fig. 12.15). Consider the most useful regions for auscultation (Fig. 12.16).

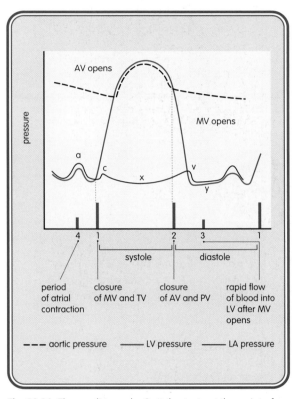

Fig. 12.14 The cardiac cycle. Systole starts at the point of closure of the mitral valve (MV)—first heart sound—when pressure in the left ventricle (LV) exceeds that of the left atrium (LA). There is a period of isovolumetric contraction before the pressure in the LV exceeds that in the aorta, at which point the aortic valve (AV) opens and blood starts to flow into the aorta. Following the onset of relaxation of the LV the aortic pressure exceeds that in the LV and the aortic valve closes—second heart sound. The ventricle continues to relax until the pressure falls below that in the filled LA and the MV opens allowing blood to flow rapidly into the LV. Atrial contraction precedes ventricular contraction, causing a presystolic accentuation of flow into the LV. (PV, pulmonary valve; TV, tricuspid valve.)

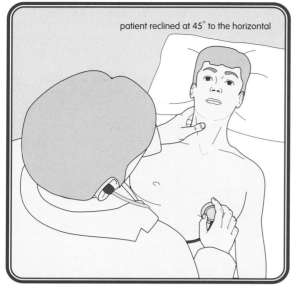

Fig. 12.15 It is essential to listen to the cardiac sounds while timing their point in the cardiac cycle by palpating the carotid pulse at the same time.

Resist the temptation to auscultate until the rest of the examination routine is completed. It is much easier to auscultate when the sounds can be put into context with the rest of the examination.

Listen in a systematic manner. In each region listen for:
- The first heart sound (immediately precedes systole).
- The second heart sound.
- Murmurs during systole.
- 'The absence of silence', usually a murmur, during diastole.
- Any extra sounds (e.g. clicks, snaps).

If a murmur is heard, characterize its features as follows:
- Volume (Fig. 12.17).
- Onset—for example presystolic, early systolic.
- Pattern—for example crescendo–decrescendo pattern of aortic stenosis.
- Termination—compare the early systolic murmur of aortic stenosis and systolic murmur of mitral regurgitation.

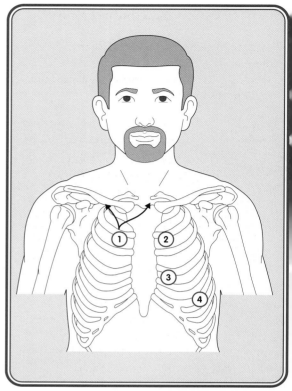

Fig. 12.16 Positions on the chest to auscultate for cardiac sounds. (1) second right intercostal space (aortic area)—mitral murmurs are very rarely audible here; if a murmur is audible, trace it towards the neck. (2) second left intercostal space (pulmonary area)—aortic regurgitation may be louder here. (3) fourth left intercostal space (tricuspid area)—especially for tricuspid regurgitation, but mitral regurgitation and aortic stenosis are often also audible here; aortic regurgitation may be loudest here. (4) Apex (mitral area)—listen specifically for mitral stenosis with the bell of the stethoscope; if a murmur is audible trace it towards the axilla.

Grading of the intensity of a cardiac murmur	
Grade	**Intensity**
I	just audible under optimal listening conditions
II	quiet
III	moderately loud
IV	loud and associated with a thrill
V	very loud
VI	audible without the aid of a stethoscope

Fig. 12.17 Grading of the intensity of a cardiac murmur.

- Pitch—for example low-pitched murmur of mitral stenosis.
- Location—where is it heard, and where is it most audible?
- Radiation—for example mitral regurgitation murmur radiating to the axilla.

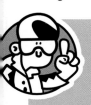

Diastolic murmurs are often difficult to hear. Listen specifically for the 'absence of silence' in diastole. Certain manoeuvres (see below) need to be performed to augment the sounds.

To elicit aortic regurgitation, sit the patient forward and listen over the right second intercostal space and left sternal edge (LSE) in fixed expiration using the diaphragm of the stethoscope. To elicit mitral stenosis, role the patient into a left lateral position and listen over the apex in fixed expiration using the bell of the stethoscope. Mild exertion may accentuate the murmur.

The different heart sounds are illustrated in Fig. 12.18.

AORTIC STENOSIS

Diagnosing the pathology

The features of aortic stenosis are illustrated in Fig. 12.19.

The murmur needs to be distinguished from the ejection systolic murmurs associated with:

- Aortic sclerosis—this is common, the patient is usually elderly, and there are no haemodynamic effects.
- Bicuspid aortic valve—this is a common cause of an ejection systolic murmur in an asymptomatic young person.
- Subvalvular aortic stenosis—there is no ejection click.
- Pulmonary stenosis—this is rare and the murmur is loudest in left 2nd intercostal space.
- Atrial septal defect—here there is a pulmonary flow murmur, fixed splitting of the second heart sound and an associated tricuspid flow murmur.

Significance of different cardiac sounds		
Audible heart sounds	**Timing**	**Cause**
first heart sound	immediately presystolic	closure of mitral and tricuspid valves
second heart sound	end of systole	closure of aortic and pulmonary valves
third heart sound	early diastole	corresponds to period of rapid ventricular filling; normal in young fit people; associated with impaired LV function (especially raised end-diastolic pressure) (low-pitched, best heard at apex)
fourth heart sound	immediately presystolic	atrial systole; associated with non-compliant LV (e.g. hypertension); best heard with bell at apex
ejection click	early systole	opening of stenotic aortic valve
opening snap	early diastole	opening of abnormal tricuspid valve and especially mitral valve in mitral stenosis (well-defined short, high-pitched sound best heard with diaphragm at left sternal edge)
pericardial rub	systole and diastole	inflamed pericardium; coarse grating sound (like walking on fresh snow); accentuated by leaning patient forwards; may be very localized

Fig. 12.18 Significance of different cardiac sounds. (LV, left ventricle.)

Features of aortic stenosis	
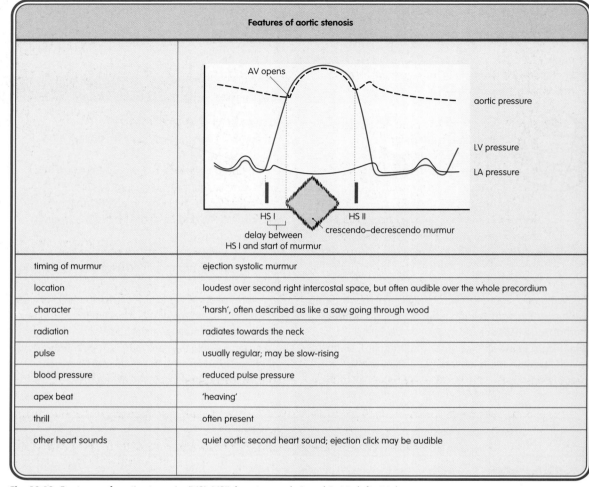	
timing of murmur	ejection systolic murmur
location	loudest over second right intercostal space, but often audible over the whole precordium
character	'harsh', often described as like a saw going through wood
radiation	radiates towards the neck
pulse	usually regular; may be slow-rising
blood pressure	reduced pulse pressure
apex beat	'heaving'
thrill	often present
other heart sounds	quiet aortic second heart sound; ejection click may be audible

Fig. 12.19 Features of aortic stenosis. (HSI, HSII, heart sounds 1 and 2; LA, left atrial; LV, left ventricular; AV, aortic valve.)

Assessing severity

Features suggestive of significant aortic stenosis include:
- Slow-rising pulse.
- Narrow pulse pressure.
- Displaced apex beat (suggestive of decompensation, unless there is associated aortic regurgitation).

Aetiology

The most common causes include:
- Degenerative disease—most common cause.
- Congenital anomaly.
- Rheumatic disease—now less common; look for associated valve pathology.

AORTIC REGURGITATION

Diagnosing the pathology

Aortic regurgitation is associated with a diastolic murmur, but there are other clues that indicate the presence of aortic regurgitation (Fig. 12.20).

The murmur of aortic regurgitation is often subtle. A specific attempt should always be made to listen for it. Sit the patient forward and listen with the diaphragm of the stethoscope in fixed expiration. Listen for the 'absence of silence' in diastole.

Features on systemic examination include:
- Pulse—collapsing, high volume.
- Nails—visible capillary pulsation (Quincke's sign).

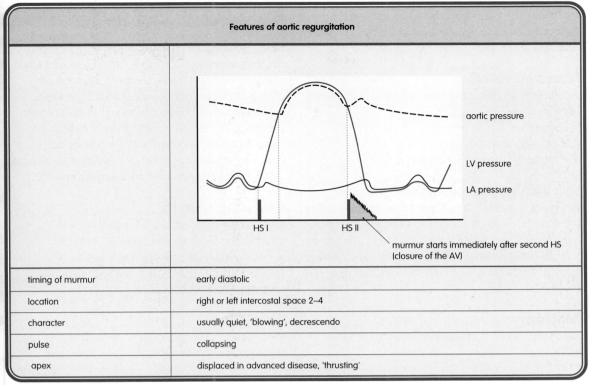

Features of aortic regurgitation	
timing of murmur	early diastolic
location	right or left intercostal space 2–4
character	usually quiet, 'blowing', decrescendo
pulse	collapsing
apex	displaced in advanced disease, 'thrusting'

Fig. 12.20 Features of aortic regurgitation.

- Neck—head nods with each systole (de Musset's sign); vigorous arterial pulsation in neck (Corrigan's sign).
- Blood pressure—wide pulse pressure.
- Apex—displaced (due to volume overload—ominous sign), thrusting.
- Peripheral pulse—diastolic murmur over lightly compressed femoral artery (Duroziez's sign).

Assessing severity

Features suggestive of severe disease include evidence of cardiac dilatation and signs of left heart failure.

Aetiology

Clues to the underlying pathology may be found as follows:

- Look at posture and arthropathy—ankylosing spondylitis.
- Look at eyes—Argyll Robertson pupils associated with syphilitic aortitis.
- Look for high-arched palate, hypermobility, arachnodactyly—Marfan's syndrome.
- Check for other valve lesions—rheumatic fever, infective endocarditis.

Austin Flint murmurs – due to a regurgitant jet of aortic regurgitation impinging on the anterior mitral leaflet – are loved by examiners! The murmur mimics that of mitral stenosis occurring in mid-diastole.

MITRAL STENOSIS

Diagnosing the pathology

A particularly high index of suspicion should be raised in a patient with atrial fibrillation. Look for the classical mitral facies (cyanotic discolouration of the cheeks), and a tapping apex beat. The murmur is often very soft and an attempt should always be made specifically to elicit it—lean the patient on the left side, and listen with the bell of the stethoscope in fixed expiration. It may be necessary to accentuate the murmur by exercise. The features of the murmur are illustrated in Fig. 12.21.

Assessing severity

Look for features of left atrial overload and consequent left heart failure, for example:

- Cyanosis.
- Pulmonary oedema.
- Hypotension (reduced cardiac output).

Look for features of right heart failure (raised JVP, peripheral oedema, left parasternal heave due to right ventricular hypertrophy). Atrial fibrillation occurs later in the natural history of the disease. The opening snap or onset of the murmur is closer to the second heart sound in severe disease as left atrial pressure is raised.

Aetiology

Rheumatic heart disease is by far the most common cause.

MITRAL REGURGITATION

Diagnosing the pathology

Mitral regurgitation is commonly heard, and produces a pansystolic murmur. It may be due to a number of different disease processes. Clues may be obtained before auscultation by the presence of atrial fibrillation (commonly occurs, but atrial fibrillation is more characteristically associated with mitral stenosis), a displaced thrusting apex beat, and occasionally a systolic thrill. Features of the murmur are illustrated in Fig. 12.22.

Assessing severity

It is often difficult to assess the severity clinically, but a third heart sound and a mid-diastolic mitral flow murmur may be detected in severe disease. The severity is usually assessed by the symptoms and haemodynamic consequences.

Aetiology

Mitral regurgitation may occur in any process that causes left ventricular dilatation and consequent

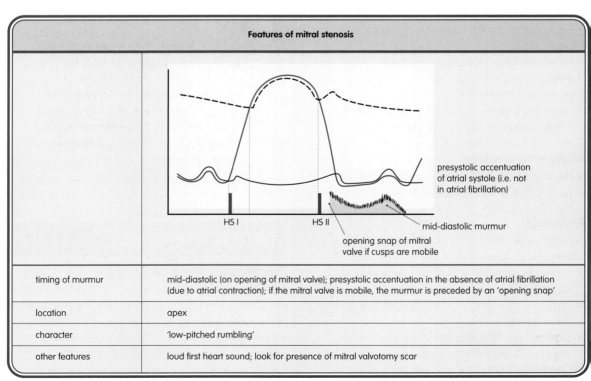

	Features of mitral stenosis
timing of murmur	mid-diastolic (on opening of mitral valve); presystolic accentuation in the absence of atrial fibrillation (due to atrial contraction); if the mitral valve is mobile, the murmur is preceded by an 'opening snap'
location	apex
character	'low-pitched rumbling'
other features	loud first heart sound; look for presence of mitral valvotomy scar

Fig. 12.21 Features of mitral stenosis.

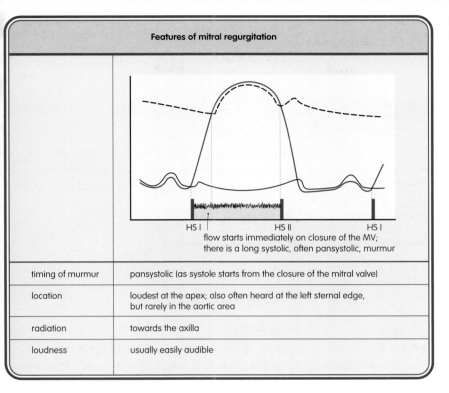

Features of mitral regurgitation

HS I | HS II | HS I

flow starts immediately on closure of the MV;
there is a long systolic, often pansystolic, murmur

timing of murmur	pansystolic (as systole starts from the closure of the mitral valve)
location	loudest at the apex; also often heard at the left sternal edge, but rarely in the aortic area
radiation	towards the axilla
loudness	usually easily audible

Fig. 12.22 Features of mitral regurgitation. (HS, heart sound; MV, mitral valve.)

stretching of the mitral valve annulus, as well as valvular pathology. The most common causes are:
- Ischaemic heart disease—by far the most common cause.
- Rheumatic heart disease—relatively common in elderly patients, but now a rare disease in the UK; often associated with mitral stenosis.
- Infective endocarditis—look for peripheral stigmata.
- Papillary muscle rupture—especially after myocardial infarction.
- Mitral valve prolapse—common and due to ballooning of the posterior leaflet into the left atrium; it is associated with a mid-systolic click and late systolic murmur.

TRICUSPID REGURGITATION

Diagnosing the pathology
Tricuspid regurgitation can often be recognized from the end of the bed by the observant examiner. It is usually due to primary left heart disease and secondary right ventricular pressure overload, so the signs may be due to a mixture of pathologies.

The jugular venous waveform shows characteristic giant v waves, and may cause oscillation of the ear lobes if the venous pressure is high enough. The patient often has signs of right heart failure with peripheral oedema and occasionally ascites. If tricuspid regurgitation is suspected, the liver should be palpated bimanually for pulsatile hepatomegaly. In addition, the underlying cause should be sought.

The murmur resembles that of mitral regurgitation in many respects (Fig. 12.23).

Assessing severity
Look for features of right-sided heart failure.

Aetiology
Tricuspid regurgitation usually results from right ventricular overload. The more common conditions predisposing to this are:
- Mitral valve disease.
- Cor pulmonale.
- Right ventricular myocardial infarction.

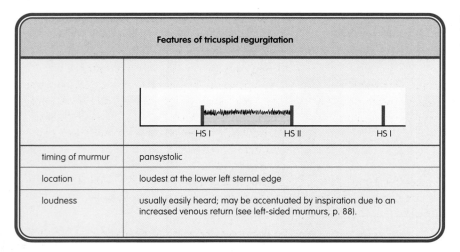

Fig. 12.23 Features of tricuspid regurgitation. (HS, heart sound.)

	Features of tricuspid regurgitation
timing of murmur	pansystolic
location	loudest at the lower left sternal edge
loudness	usually easily heard; may be accentuated by inspiration due to an increased venous return (see left-sided murmurs, p. 88).

Primary tricuspid regurgitation may occur in:
- Rheumatic fever—rarely an isolated valve lesion.
- Infective endocarditis—especially in drug addicts (look for needle marks).
- Carcinoid syndrome—look for hepatomegaly, flushing, signs of pulmonary stenosis.

INFECTIVE ENDOCARDITIS

Infective endocarditis may affect any of the heart valves. It often presents in a non-specific manner and should be suspected in all patients with newly diagnosed valvular pathology or those with pre-existing valvular disease who develop pyrexia and malaise or a change in murmur.

Valvular pathology and severity
Define the valvular lesions and the haemodynamic consequences by a thorough cardiovascular examination.

Peripheral stigmata suggesting endocarditis
A complete systemic examination is essential as manifestations may arise from many systems. Features on systemic examination include the following.

Pyrexia
Fever is almost universal in infective endocarditis. However, it is often low grade and a single temperature reading may be normal. It is very important to follow the progression of fever through the course of the illness as a marker of successful therapy.

Nails
There are multiple stigmata of infective endocarditis in the hands. Many of these arise from an associated vasculitis. The following signs may be detected in the nails (do not forget to examine the toes!):
- Splinter haemorrhages. These are a non-specific finding, but common. They are suggestive of a vasculitic process. Although the presence is not specific for vasculitis, the occurrence of new splinter haemorrhages developing in the context of a new murmur and fever is highly suggestive of infective endocarditis.
- Nailfold infarcts. These are also suggestive of a vasculitic process. They are more specific, but less common than splinter haemorrhages.
- Clubbing. A late sign and hopefully not present!

Hands
Vasculitic signs may also be detected in the hands:
- Osler's nodes. Do not forget the four Ps (painful, purple, papules on the pulps) of the fingers—this is rare, but enjoyed by examiners!

- Janeway lesions. These are rare transient macular patches on the palms.

Eyes

Fundoscopy is essential (especially in the exam setting). Look for Roth's spots, which are characteristic flame-shaped haemorrhages on the retina with white centres.

Splenomegaly

Splenomegaly is usually barely palpable, if at all. There is little correlation with the duration or severity of the disease.

Haematuria

An immune complex nephritis is a common feature. Remember that urinalysis is part of the examination. Haematuria usually clears with successful antibiotic therapy. Occasionally confusion may arise as the long-term antibiotic therapy may precipitate interstitial nephritis (e.g. penicillins) or be nephrotoxic (e.g. gentamicin).

Neurological signs

Endocarditis may present with neurological signs due to septic emboli in the brain. The elderly may present non-specifically with confusion.

Aetiology

Risk factors for infection may be elicited from the examination:

- Right-sided valve lesions—especially in intravenous drug abusers (*Staphylococcus aureus* and fungal disease more likely in this group of patients).
- Underlying valve lesion—usually present; *Streptococcus viridans* is the most common agent; the most common predisposing valvular lesions are mitral and aortic valve disease, ventricular septal defect (VSD), patent ductus arteriosus (PDA), and coarctation of the aorta.
- Prosthetic valve.
- Poor dental hygiene—often the mouth is the primary portal of entry.

HEART FAILURE

A diagnosis of heart failure is inadequate. An attempt must be made to assess its severity, functional impact, and aetiology.

Establishing the diagnosis and differentiating the features of right and left heart failure

Clues from the systemic examination are shown in Fig. 12.24. High-output cardiac failure may also occur in conditions such as thyrotoxicosis or Paget's disease. (Fig. 12.25). Not all of the features may be present and they depend upon the severity and underlying cause. Often left and right heart failure coexist.

Assessment of severity is usually dependent upon the history and the functional limitation imposed on the patient.

Signs of right and left heart failure	
Right heart failure	**Left heart failure**
raised jugular venous pressure	third heart sound
peripheral oedema	displaced apex beat (if volume overload)
ascites	pulmonary oedema
hepatomegaly	tachycardia
left parasternal heave	cyanosis
cyanosis	cool, sweaty, pale skin (low-output state)
tricuspid regurgitation	mitral regurgitation (due to volume overload of left ventricle)

Fig. 12.24 Signs of right and left heart failure.

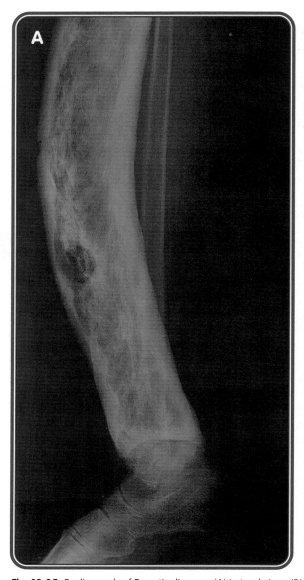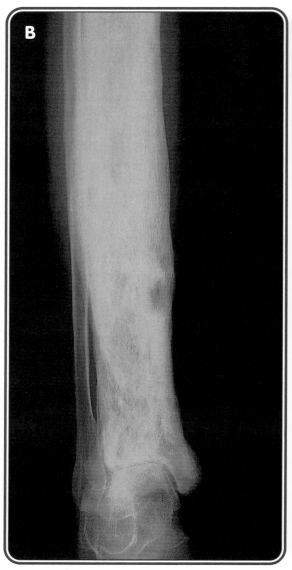

Fig. 12.25 Radiograph of Paget's disease. (A) Lateral view. (B) Antero-posterior (A-P) view. Paget's disease occasionally causes high-output cardiac failure. Note the bowing of the tibia and widespread sclerosis with coarse trabeculae.

Aetiology

The principal causes of heart failure are:
- Impaired myocardial contractility.
- Arrhythmia.
- Volume overload.
- Pressure overload.
- Impaired filling.

Features of these conditions are illustrated in Fig. 12.26.

MYOCARDIAL INFARCTION

Often, there are no specific physical signs following a myocardial infarction (MI), but the physical examination can reveal complications and guide management, both in the acute setting and in the ensuing period.

Inspection

A quick visual inspection may reveal signs of pain or

Features of different types of heart failure on systemic examination.	
Cause of heart failure	**Features**
impaired myocardial contractility ischaemic heart disease	most common cause; may present as right, left, or biventricular failure; look for features to suggest other vascular disease (e.g. carotid bruits, signs of hypertension, etc.)
cardiomyopathy	look for systemic disease (e.g. amyloid, etc.)
myocarditis	look for signs of systemic infection; tachycardia is often a prominent feature; listen for associated pericardial rub
arrhythmia	common; often exacerbates underlying heart disease; may be able to detect arrhythmia from the pulse; aim to distinguish a primary arrhythmia from one consequent on poor myocardial perfusion
volume overload aortic regurgitation mitral regurgitation tricuspid regurgitation	look for signs of an underlying valvular defect; for left-sided lesions, identify a displaced apex beat
pressure overload hypertension aortic stenosis pulmonary embolus	slow-rising pulse; narrow pulse pressure; sustained apex beat right-sided signs associated with hypotension
impaired ventricular filling mitral stenosis cardiac tamponade restrictive cardiomyopathy	right heart failure; pulsus paradoxus; note jugular waveform

Fig. 12.26 Features of different types of heart failure on systemic examination.

discomfort, necessitating better analgesic control. Assess peripheral perfusion—a cold, sweaty, cyanosed, pale patient suggests shock.

Complications
Always check for the presence of complications such as left or right heart failure and the presence of arrhythmias.

Left heart failure
Look for features of left heart failure, such as:
- Signs of poor peripheral perfusion (impaired cardiac output).
- Low-volume pulse.
- Inspiratory crepitations at the lung bases.
- Third heart sound.
- Dyspnoea.

These signs may indicate that the patient will not tolerate β-blockade or may benefit from diuretics and angiotensin-converting enzyme (ACE) inhibitors.

Right heart failure
It is very important to recognize the patient with a right ventricular infarction. A disproportionately raised JVP in association with very poor peripheral perfusion, hypotension, and ECG signs are characteristic. Fluid balance in these patients is critical and demands central monitoring to assess left atrial filling pressure.

Arrhythmia
Check the pulse carefully. Usually there is a mild tachycardia. The presence of a bradycardia suggests an inferior-wall MI. The pulse may give clues to an underlying rhythm disturbance, for example:
- Heart block—especially following anterior-wall MI.
- Atrial fibrillation—common.
- Ventricular extrasystoles.

95

These should be confirmed as the patient will have continuous ECG recording.

Subsequent examination

Once patients are on the ward, they should be examined at least daily. Particular features to assess include:

- Pulse rate (β-blocker, primary cardiac rhythm disturbance). (e.g. excessive bradycardia induced by β-blocker, primary cardiac rhythm disturbance such as atrial fibrillation or ventrical tachycardia)
- Blood pressure (e.g. cardiogenic shock, primary hypertension, or new therapy with β-blocker or ACE inhibitor may cause hypertension).
- Signs of heart failure.
- Murmurs—especially that of mitral regurgitation due to papillary muscle rupture and the long systolic murmur of ventricular septal defect.

- Pericardial rub.
- Psychological rehabilitation—often, the greatest morbidity on discharge from hospital is psychological; this should be recognized, and treated early by appropriate education and reassurance.
- Signs of deep vein thrombosis—especially if there has been prolonged bed rest.

In the presence of shock and signs of right heart failure, always consider the presence of a posterior infarct, which may be subtle on the ECG.

13. Respiratory Examination

EXAMINATION ROUTINE

Patient exposure and position

The patient should be exposed to the waist in a similar fashion to exposure for the cardiovascular examination (see p. 79), and seated comfortably on a couch, inclined at 45 degrees to the horizontal in a well-lit room.

General inspection

This should be performed systematically. As with other systems, think about which features you are looking for before inspection. It is convenient to look first at the patient generally, and then to inspect specific features from the head downwards. This process need take only a few seconds.

General features

Note the following features:
- Age and sex of the patient.
- General health and body habitus.
- Comfort at rest. For example, how easily can the patient climb onto the examination couch?
- Respiratory rate. This is an important, often inadequately elicited, sign.
- General environment. For example, in a hospital, look on the bedside cabinet for sputum pots, nebulizers, inhalers, peak flow charts.

Head

Look for evidence of:
- Central cyanosis (requires at least 5 g/dL deoxygenated haemoglobin).
- Plethora (e.g. from secondary polycythaemia due to chronic hypoxia).
- Cigarette staining of hair and smell of cigarettes.

Chest

Note the presence of :
- Scars (Fig. 13.1)
- Breathing pattern (e.g. use of accessory muscles—sternomastoid, intercostals, abdominal, etc.)

- Chest wall deformity (e.g. pectus excavatum).
- Asymmetry (e.g. due to previous tuberculosis causing upper lobe fibrosis).
- Obvious tracheal deviation.

Specific examination

A more detailed systematic examination can now begin.

Hands

In particular look for the presence of:
- Clubbing (see p. 80).
- Peripheral cyanosis—if present, check for central cyanosis.
- Cigarette staining of nails and fingers.

Blood pressure and arterial pulse

A quick assessment of the pulse rate and blood pressure is useful. A hyperdynamic circulation may occur in carbon dioxide retention. In the presence of asthma, quantify pulsus paradoxus (see p. 84).

Head

An assessment should include specific inspection of:
- Eyes—to reveal for example Horner's syndrome (due to carcinoma of bronchus), jaundice, conjunctival pallor.
- Mouth—for example tongue and mucous membranes may be cyanosed.

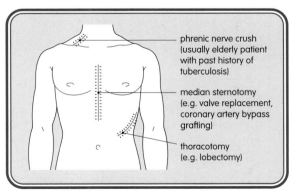

phrenic nerve crush (usually elderly patient with past history of tuberculosis)

median sternotomy (e.g. valve replacement, coronary artery bypass grafting)

thoracotomy (e.g. lobectomy)

Fig. 13.1 Scars related to the respiratory system.

Neck
Lymphadenopathy
Examine the cervical and supraclavicular lymph nodes. It may be easier to defer this part of the examination until the patient is sitting forward so that palpation can be performed from the rear.

Jugular venous pressure and waveform
A brief assessment may indicate the presence of cor pulmonale or superior vena cava obstruction.

Tracheal position
Remember that this part of the examination is slightly uncomfortable (Fig. 13.2). The trachea may be shifted by pathology outside the chest (e.g. thyroid enlargement). Mediastinal position can also be assessed by determining the position of the apex beat.

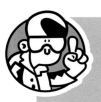

The tracheal position is often neglected by students, but this sign is of fundamental importance as it indicates the presence of a focal chest expanding (e.g. tension pneumothorax, massive pleural effusion) or constricting process (fibrosis, lung collapse).

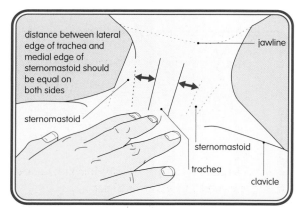

Fig. 13.2 Examination technique for assessing tracheal position. Place two fingers on either side of the trachea and judge the distance between the fingers and the sternomastoid tendons.

Chest
Although the routine for chest examination is straightforward, the interpretation of signs requires experience as very often they reflect only a 'qualitative' difference from the normal state. An appreciation of the range of normality demands practice! There are no short cuts! It is invaluable to have a more experienced observer who can provide constructive criticism of your approach and interpretation of signs with you while you are examining the patient.

Very few chest pathologies are manifest as a single abnormal sign. Rather, a constellation of signs needs to be interpreted in context and then integrated. The successful examiner will be constantly analysing the elicited signs and refining a differential diagnosis, anticipating how the next sign may modify the assessment. This highlights the importance of adopting an active approach to the examination. Inspiration rarely comes at the *end* of the examination!

It is a matter of preference whether the whole process is performed on the front of the chest and then the back, or whether each component of the examination is completed for the whole chest in turn, but the former is more comfortable for the patient and is preferred.

Resist the temptation to auscultate too early. Always examine the chest in the following standard order:
- **Inspection.**
- **Palpation.**
- **Percussion.**
- **Auscultation.**

Inspection
If tracheal shift is noted, look more closely for asymmetry, especially scalloping below the clavicles suggesting loss of volume of the upper lobe.

Palpation
There are three main components to this section:
- Assessment of mediastinal position.
- Assessment of chest expansion.
- Tactile vocal fremitus (TVF). (Vocal resonance will also be discussed in this section for ease of explanation.)

Assessment of mediastinal position: If the trachea is deviated, the position of the lower mediastinum can be assessed by determining the position of the apex beat. Exclude dextrocardia (Kartagener's syndrome, which is very rare, but enjoyed by examiners!).

Chest expansion: Assess the degree and symmetry of chest expansion. Expansion should be assessed in the infraclavicular, costal margin, and lower rib region posteriorly (Fig. 13.3).

If there is unilateral chest pathology, the side of the chest with reduced expansion always indicates the side of the pathology.

Tactile vocal fremitus: Place the medial aspect of the hand on the chest wall and ask the patient to make a resonant sound (e.g. say 'ninety nine'). The sound waves are transmitted as low-frequency vibrations, which are palpable. Different regions of the chest should be examined systematically, in particular comparing symmetry of the two sides. Make an attempt to define abnormalities in the upper, middle, and lower lobes. This requires an awareness of the surface markings of these lobes (Fig. 13.4).

Vocal resonance: This is included here as it is complementary to TVF. Place the stethoscope on the chest wall and ask the patient to whisper 'one, two, three'. The distinct sounds are not normally well defined, but a resonant sound is detectable as the sound waves are altered by transmission through the airways and chest wall. Once again, different regions should be examined systematically, comparing symmetry. Increased vocal resonance is termed whispering pectoriloquy.

The degree of TVF or vocal resonance is dependent upon the transmission of sound waves to the chest wall from the large bronchi. It is therefore dependent upon the volume of sound generated and the conductivity of the lungs, which is dependent upon how close the stethoscope is to a large bronchus. It is:

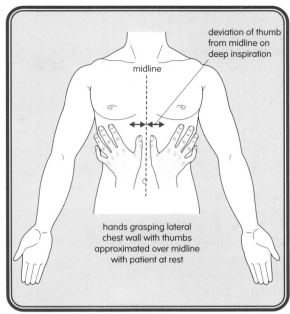

deviation of thumb from midline on deep inspiration

midline

hands grasping lateral chest wall with thumbs approximated over midline with patient at rest

Fig. 13.3 Examination of chest expansion. The primary objective is to assess symmetry. Assess expansion in the upper, lower, and middle regions of the chest. Place hands around the lateral chest wall and approximate the thumbs in the midline (but not resting on the chest). Ask the patient to take a deep breath and observe the displacement of the thumbs from the midline.

- Increased in consolidation or lung collapse with a patent airway.
- Decreased in pleural effusion, pneumothorax, or collapse with an obstructed bronchus.

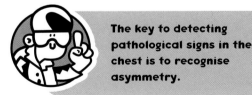
The key to detecting pathological signs in the chest is to recognise asymmetry.

Percussion

Percussion is performed by placing the middle or index finger of one hand on the chest wall and hyperexpanding the proximal and distal interphalangeal joints so that the middle phalanx is closely opposed to the chest wall, and tapping it with the opposite index finger. This action should come from

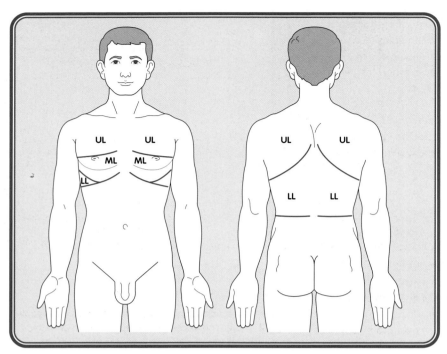

Fig. 13.4 Surface markings of the individual lobes (UL, upper lobe; ML, middle lobe; LL, lower lobe) of the lungs. Make an attempt to assess percussion, vocal fremitus, and auscultation in each region so that any pathology can be localized to a particular lobe.

the wrist, rather than being a hammering action, and be just heavy enough to detect resonance. The percussing finger should be rapidly withdrawn after striking. Resonance is felt, just as much as it is heard. Percussion should be performed systematically as for TVF. Findings may include:

- Hyperresonance of the percussion note. This is often difficult to elicit, but is present if there is more air than normal in the chest cavity (e.g. pneumothorax, emphysema).
- A dull percussion note. This occurs if the lung tissue is replaced by solid material (e.g. consolidation) or if solid material is present between the chest wall and the lung (e.g. pleural effusion, pleural thickening).

In practice, it is easier to detect decreased or absent tactile vocal fremitus and increased vocal resonance from the normal state. Hence, the two signs complement each other.

Auscultation

Breath sounds are produced by turbulent airflow, and transmitted through the airways, lung parenchyma, pleurae, and chest wall. Changes in any of these structures can alter the sounds heard.

Auscultation is usually performed with the diaphragm of the stethoscope as the patient breathes fairly deeply. It is important to compare findings on the two sides.

The aim of auscultation is to define:

- The quality of the breath sounds (Fig. 13.5).
- The presence of added sounds—as with cardiac murmurs, characterize the quality, volume, and timing.
- Vocal resonance (see above).

Added sounds should be characterized systematically. Note the presence of the following sounds.

Crackles (crepitations): These may be caused by secretions in the larger airways (e.g. in bronchitis, pneumonia, bronchiectasis). They are usually present throughout inspiration and may clear on coughing. Alternatively, reopening of occluded small airways during the later part of inspiration occurs in parenchymal disease (e.g. fibrosis, interstitial oedema). Coughing will then have no effect.

Wheezes (rhonchi): These have a musical quality and

Description of the quality of breath sounds		
Breath sounds	**Features**	**Examples**
vesicular breathing	progressively louder during inspiration, merging into expiratory phase with rapid fading in intensity	normal pattern
bronchial breathing	laryngeal sounds transmitted efficiently to chest wall if lung substance becomes uniform and more solid—blowing quality; pause between inspiratory and expiratory phases; expiratory phase as long as inspiratory phase	consolidation; collapse with patent bronchus; fibrosis
diminished volume	impaired conduction due to increased pleural/chest wall thickness or increased air acting as poor conductor	pleural effusion; pleural thickening; obesity; emphysema; pneumothorax

Fig. 13.5 Description of the quality of breath sounds.

usually result from narrowing of the bronchi due to oedema, spasm, tumour, secretions. They occur in:
- Asthma—polyphonic, mainly expiratory, diffuse.
- Bronchitis—may clear on coughing, may have an inspiratory component.
- Fixed obstruction—monophonic (e.g. due to bronchial carcinoma).

Pleural rub: This sound is due to friction between the visceral and parietal pleurae in inflammatory conditions (pleurisy). It is often described as the sound of walking on crisp, newly fallen snow.

Summary

At the end of the respiratory examination, it is important to take time to reflect on your findings. Remember that few lung pathologies have a single pathognomonic feature and that abnormalities are often a matter of qualitative judgement of deviation from normality rather than the simple presence or absence of a sign. The key to a successful examination is to be attentive and open to differential diagnoses from the start, so that physical signs can be anticipated rather than taking you by surprise.

PLEURAL EFFUSION

Diagnosing the pathology

The physical signs can be anticipated from a basic appreciation of the pathology (Fig. 13.6).

Assessing severity

Analyse the significance of physical signs, for example:
- How high up the chest can percussion be demonstrated to be stony dull?
- Define the level of decreased breath sounds and reduced TVF.
- How dyspnoeic is the patient? (This may be altered by coexisting pathology and speed of onset.)
- Is the trachea shifted away from the effusion?

Aetiology

Look for clues in the systemic examination:
- Palpable supraclavicular and/or axillary lymphadenopathy—malignancy.
- Hepatomegaly—secondary malignancy.
- Peripheral oedema—hypoalbuminaemia, heart failure.
- Third heart sound—left heart failure.

Consider the more common causes of pleural effusion (Fig. 13.7).

PNEUMOTHORAX

Diagnosing the pathology

A small pneumothorax can be hard to identify, but index of suspicion should be high in tall, thin, young adults with sudden-onset pleuritic chest pain and dyspnoea. The basic clinical signs can be elucidated from basic principles (Fig. 13.8).

101

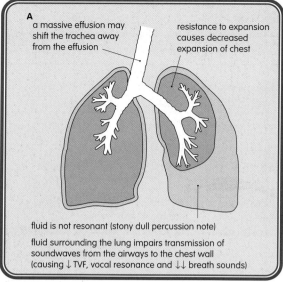

A

a massive effusion may shift the trachea away from the effusion

resistance to expansion causes decreased expansion of chest

fluid is not resonant (stony dull percussion note)

fluid surrounding the lung impairs transmission of soundwaves from the airways to the chest wall (causing ↓TVF, vocal resonance and ↓↓ breath sounds)

Fig. 13.6 (A) Physical signs of a pleural effusion. (B) Radiograph of a massive left pleural effusion. Note the tracheal deviation to the right. (TVF, tactile vocal fremitus.)

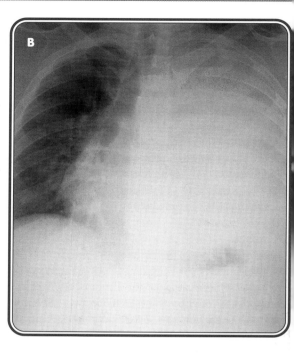

B

Common causes of a pleural effusion	
Transudates	**Exudates**
left heart failure*	infection* (pneumonia, tuberculosis, empyema, etc.)
hypoalbuminuric states* (e.g. nephrotic syndrome, liver failure)	malignancy* (primary bronchial or metastatic)
	pulmonary infarction*
fluid overload in renal failure	subphrenic abscess
hypothyroidism	
	pancreatitis
Meigs's syndrome (right pleural effusion in association with ovarian fibroma)	collagen vascular disease (e.g. rheumatoid arthritis)
	haemothorax

Fig. 13.7 Common causes of a pleural effusion. The more common causes are marked with an asterisk.

Assessing severity

Most pneumothoraces do not cause haemodynamic compromise, but it is important to recognize a tension pneumothorax. This produces deviation of the trachea and is a medical emergency.

A tension pneumothorax is a medical emergency and should be identified and treated before requesting a radiograph.

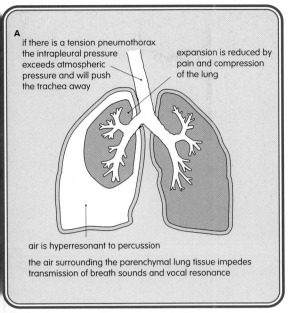

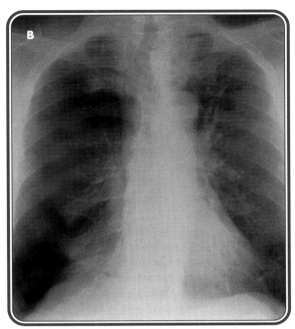

Fig. 13.8 (A) Physical signs of pneumothorax.
B) Radiograph of a right pneumothorax.

Within image A:

A

if there is a tension pneumothorax
the intrapleural pressure
exceeds atmospheric
pressure and will push
the trachea away

expansion is reduced by
pain and compression
of the lung

air is hyperresonant to percussion

the air surrounding the parenchymal lung tissue impedes
transmission of breath sounds and vocal resonance

Aetiology

Most spontaneous pneumothoraces occur in previously
fit young adults and are idiopathic. Look for underlying
lung disease that may have precipitated the event.
Consider the three major groups of precipitating
pathologies, which are:

- Underlying medical disease (e.g. asthma,
  emphysema and bullae, carcinoma, tuberculosis).
- Iatrogenic (e.g. after central venous line insertion,
  especially subclavian line, intubated patient with
  positive pressure ventilation, after pleural aspiration
  or biopsy).
- Trauma (e.g. fractured ribs, look for surgical
  emphysema).

LUNG COLLAPSE

Diagnosing the pathology

Lung collapse may occur with a patent or occluded
bronchus. The physical signs will differ and may
depend upon severity and underlying cause (Figs 13.9
and 13.10).

Aetiology

Consider the more common causes of collapse.

Extrinsic compression

The most common cause of lung collapse is lymph node
compression due to tumour or tuberculosis.

Intrinsic obstruction

Intraluminal obstruction may occlude the airway and
cause distal collapse. The more common causes include:

- Tumours—look for clubbing.
- Retained secretions—postoperative, debilitated
  patients.
- Inhaled foreign body—usually apparent from history,
  especially right lower lobe—a medical emergency!
- Bronchial cast or plug—for example, due to
  aspergillosis, blood clot.

CONSOLIDATION

Diagnosing the pathology

Consolidation implies replacement of air in the acini with
fluid or solid material. The lung parenchyma is heavy

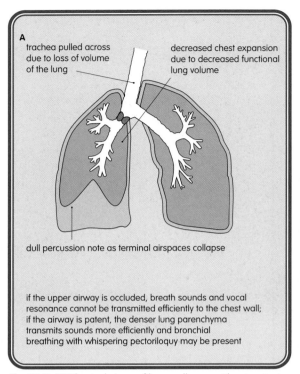

A

trachea pulled across due to loss of volume of the lung

decreased chest expansion due to decreased functional lung volume

dull percussion note as terminal airspaces collapse

if the upper airway is occluded, breath sounds and vocal resonance cannot be transmitted efficiently to the chest wall; if the airway is patent, the denser lung parenchyma transmits sounds more efficiently and bronchial breathing with whispering pectoriloquy may be present

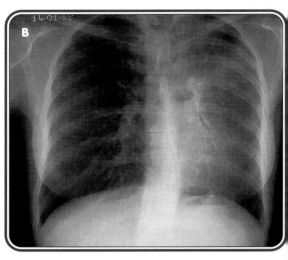

B

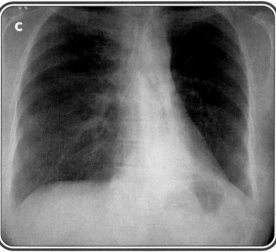

C

Fig. 13.9 (A) Physical signs of lung collapse without patent upper airways. (B) Radiograph of left upper lobe collapse: loss of lung volume is indicated by deviation of the trachea to the left, mediastinal shift to the left, and loss of volume of the left lung; in addition, note the classic veil-like opacification over the left lung. (C) Radiograph of left lower lobe collapse: note the raised left hemidiaphragm, mediastinal shift to the left, loss of volume and hypertranslucency of the left lung, and depressed left hilum indicating loss of lung volume, in association with a change in density behind the heart shadow.

Fig. 13.10 Physical signs of lung collapse with and without patent upper airways. (TVF, tactile vocal fremitus.)

Physical signs of lung collapse with and without patent upper airways		
Sign	**Patent upper airway**	**Obstructed bronchus**
expansion	always reduced on side of lesion	always reduced on side of lesion
trachea	deviated to side of collapse, especially upper lobe collapse	deviated to side of collapse, especially upper lobe collapse
percussion	dull	dull
TVF	usually normal or increased	decreased or absent
vocal resonance	whispering pectoriloquy	—
breath sounds	increased; bronchial breathing	absent or decreased

and stiff, but transmits sound waves to the chest wall more efficiently. In addition, the lower airways often collapse during expiration, but may open explosively during inspiration when negative intrathoracic pressure is generated, producing crackles (Fig. 13.11).

Aetiology

The important causes of consolidation include:

- Pneumonia—most common cause, especially if in classical lobar distribution.
- Pulmonary oedema—may be cardiogenic or non-cardiogenic (e.g. adult respiratory distress syndrome [ARDS], hypoproteinaemia).
- Pulmonary haemorrhage—for example due to pulmonary vasculitis.
- Aspiration.
- Neoplasms—for example alveolar cell carcinoma.
- Alveolar proteinosis—rare.

Look for systemic clues of the aetiology:

- Fever, green sputum in sputum pot—pneumonia.
- Third heart sound, mitral murmurs, peripheral oedema—cardiogenic.
- Nailfold infarcts, livedo reticularis, splinter haemorrhages—vasculitis.

- Clubbing—underlying primary bronchial carcinoma.

Differential diagnosis

Clinically, the main differential diagnosis is between pneumonia and pulmonary oedema. This is usually apparent from the clinical setting. It is more likely to be pneumonia if the consolidation is in a lobar distribution or unilateral (especially right-sided). In addition, a pleural effusion, raised jugular venous pressure, and peripheral oedema are more common in pulmonary oedema, but not diagnostic.

LUNG FIBROSIS

Pulmonary fibrosis results in lungs that are rigid and resistant to expansion. The fibrotic disease often shrinks the lung, resulting in a constrictive process. The thicker parenchyma will, however, transmit sound waves more efficiently to the chest wall. As with other parenchymal processes, the small airways may open explosively in inspiration, causing crackles. The disease may be unilateral (e.g. tuberculosis) or bilateral (e.g. cryptogenic fibrosing alveolitis).

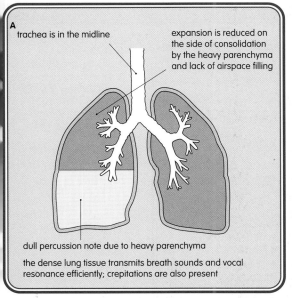

A
trachea is in the midline

expansion is reduced on the side of consolidation by the heavy parenchyma and lack of airspace filling

dull percussion note due to heavy parenchyma

the dense lung tissue transmits breath sounds and vocal resonance efficiently; crepitations are also present

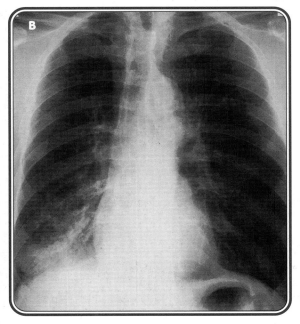

Fig. 13.11 (A) Physical signs of consolidation. (B) Radiograph of right lower lobe pneumonia.

Diagnosing the pathology

Distinguish unilateral and bilateral disease. The tracheal position is most useful as there is often coexisting pathology (Fig. 13.12).

Aetiology

The more common causes of pulmonary fibrosis are illustrated in Fig. 13.13.

INTEGRATING PHYSICAL SIGNS TO DIAGNOSE PATHOLOGY

Fig. 13.14 illustrates how the different physical signs elicited in the respiratory system can be integrated so that the basic underlying pathological cause can be identified. Remember that this is only part of the examination process. It is important to assess the severity of the pathology and its underlying cause so that specific therapy can be offered.

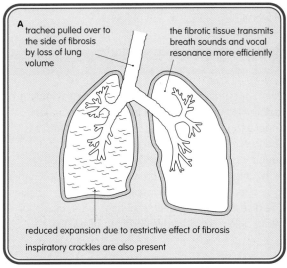

A — trachea pulled over to the side of fibrosis by loss of lung volume

the fibrotic tissue transmits breath sounds and vocal resonance more efficiently

reduced expansion due to restrictive effect of fibrosis

inspiratory crackles are also present

Fig. 13.12 (A) Physical signs of pulmonary fibrosis. (B) Radiograph of bilateral mid and lower zone pulmonary fibrosis.

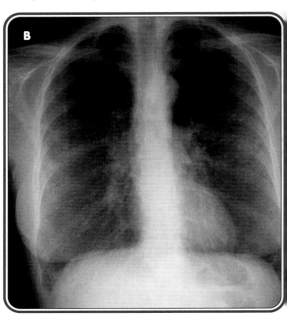

Fig. 13.13 Causes of pulmonary fibrosis. The more common causes are marked with an asterisk.

Causes of pulmonary fibrosis	
Cause	**Examples and signs**
infection*	tuberculosis (typically upper lobe)
collagen disorder	rheumatoid lung (usually basal); scleroderma
extrinsic allergic alveolitis*	especially upper lobes
sarcoidosis*	look for erythema nodosum and other stigmata
radiation	look for radiation burns
drugs	busulphan, bleomycin, etc.
cryptogenic fibrosing alveolitis	rare; begins in lower lobes; look for clubbing
asbestosis	—
ankylosing spondylitis	upper lobes; rigid back; peripheral arthritis; aortic regurgitation; etc.

The importance of assessing expansion (to reveal the side of the pathology) and tracheal position (for expanding or constricting lesions) cannot be overemphasized.

ASTHMA

A diagnosis of asthma is usually apparent from the history. The aim of the examination is to assess severity, to look for complications, and to consider precipitating factors.

Assessing severity

Use objective reproducible measures of severity and classify the attack as mild, moderate, or severe.

Remember that not all of the features need to be present in a severe attack (Fig. 13.15). The essential parameters to assess are pulse rate, pulsus paradoxus (if easily identified), respiratory rate, peak flow rate, and (in hospitals) arterial blood gas estimate.

Other features of a serious or life-threatening attack include:

- Difficulty in speaking.
- Bradycardia or hypotension.
- Exhaustion.
- Silent chest.
- Cyanosis.
- Pulsus paradoxus.

Complications

Examine for the presence of a pneumothorax. This is the main reason for radiography in hospitalized patients.

Examination findings for basic lung pathologies					
Lung pathology	Tracheal position	Percussion note	TVF/vocal resonance	Volume of breath sounds	Added sounds
pneumothorax	normal (deviated away in tension pneumothorax)	hyperresonant (often subtle)	decreased (or absent)	decreased or absent	—
consolidation	normal	dull	increased	increased (bronchial breathing)	inspiratory crackles
fibrosis	pulled towards	slightly dull	increased	increased	inspiratory crackles
pleural effusion	normal (deviated away if massive)	stony dull	reduced or absent	decreased or absent	often crackles immediately above effusion
lobar collapse (patent airway)	pulled towards	dull	increased	increased (bronchial breathing)	—
lobar collapse (occluded bronchus)	pulled towards	dull	decreased	decreased	—

Fig. 13.14 Examination findings for the basic lung pathologies. Note that this refers to unilateral lesions. The expansion is always reduced on the side of the lung pathology. (TVF, tactile vocal fremitus.)

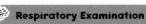

Assessment of severity of an acute asthma attack			
Feature	Mild	Moderate	Severe
pulse rate (/min)	< 100	100–110	> 110
respiratory rate (/min)	< 20	20–30	> 30
pulsus paradoxus (mmHg)	< 5	5–15	> 15
peak flow rate	> 75% predicted	50–75% predicted	< 50% predicted
arterial blood gases	PaO_2 high/normal; $PaCO_2$ low	PaO_2 normal; $PaCO_2$ low or low normal (< 5 kPa)	PaO_2 < 8 kPa; $PaCO_2$ high normal or high (> 5 kPa)

Fig. 13.15 Assessment of severity of an acute asthma attack. In the hospital setting, arterial blood gases (ABG) form part of the routine assessment. Pulsus paradoxus, if easy to elicit, is useful, but often it is difficult—it is a waste of time making an inaccurate 'best guess'.

Aetiology

Look for signs of a chest infection, which is common. In older patients with new-onset asthma, look for nasal polyps, which are also associated with aspirin sensitivity. Also inspect for features of atopy, especially in younger patients (e.g. eczema, dry skin, thinning of lateral half of eyebrows from rubbing).

 Asthma is potentially fatal. A rapid and objective assessment is essential.

LUNG CANCER

Lung cancer is the most common fatal malignancy in men, and the second in women. It can present in many ways and show many features on examination.

Inspection

Look for clues such as:
- Cachexia (common).
- Cigarette staining in hair.
- Scar from lobectomy.
- Radiotherapy burn on chest wall.

Hands

There are often signs in the hands as follows:
- Clubbing—may predate clinical diagnosis.
- Clues to smoking history—nicotine staining on nails.
- Hypertrophic pulmonary osteoarthropathy (HPOA)—pain and swelling of the wrists, especially with small-cell carcinoma.

Face

Horner's syndrome (small pupil, partial ptosis, enophthalmos, anhidrosis, due to invasion of the sympathetic ganglion T1 by direct spread) may be a feature of upper lobe disease.

Neck

Palpate for a supraclavicular lymph node. Look for features of superior vena cava obstruction (swollen face and neck, plethora, dilated veins over trunk).

Chest

Look for features of:
- Pleural effusion (common).
- Loss of lung volume due to lobar or lung collapse.

Evidence of spread
Direct spread
Examine specifically for other features of direct spread, such as:

- Pancoast's tumour—apical tumour invading the lower brachial plexus (especially C8, T1, T2) causing sensory loss, wasting, and weakness of the small muscles of the hand.
- Phrenic nerve—diaphragmatic palsy.
- Pericardium—effusion (look for features to suggest tamponade).

Metastatic spread
Examine for features of metastatic spread, for example:

- Hepatomegaly.
- Focal neurological signs due to cerebral metastases.
- Localized bony tenderness.

14. Abdominal Examination

A thorough abdominal examination is fundamental to both surgical and medical clerking, but the emphasis clearly changes according to the presenting complaint.

Patient exposure and position

Ensure good lighting. Patients should be undressed so that a view of the whole abdomen (from nipple to knees) can be obtained. Provide a blanket for warmth and modesty. Lie patients flat on the couch with a single pillow behind their head (though this may not always be possible if, for example, the patient has orthopnoea or musculoskeletal abnormalities), with arms by their side. If patients are unable to relax their abdomen fully, ask them to flex their hips to 45 degrees and knees to 90 degrees (Fig. 14.1).

The key is to have a relaxed patient. You will be able to elicit signs more easily if the patient is comfortable.

General inspection

Observe the general appearance of the patient. Time spent at this stage is invaluable. Take at least 10 seconds, making a mental checklist, for example:

- Is the patient comfortable or distressed at rest?
- Is there any obvious pain?
- Is there any cachexia, pallor, jaundice, or abnormal skin pigmentation.

A rapid but systematic survey of the patient should ensue.

Hands

Careful examination of the hands is fundamental to the abdominal examination and may yield vital clues of underlying abdominal disease.

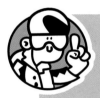

If asked to examine the abdominal system in an examination, always start by looking at the hands.

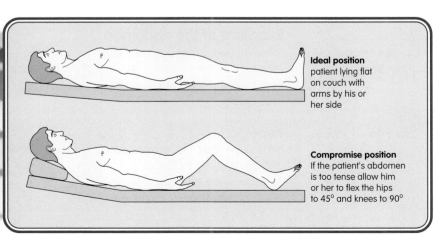

Ideal position
patient lying flat on couch with arms by his or her side

Compromise position
If the patient's abdomen is too tense allow him or her to flex the hips to 45° and knees to 90°

Fig. 14.1 Ideal position for examination of the abdomen.

Note the presence of:

- Metabolic flap (asterixis). This may indicate hepatic encephalopathy, carbon dioxide retention or uraemia.
- Signs of chronic liver disease. Inspect and palpate both hands for the presence of Dupuytren's contracture, palmar erythema, leuconychia (white nails), spider naevi, and clubbing.
- Anaemia. If the patient is profoundly anaemic, palmar skin creases may be pale. Koilonychia (spoon-shaped nails) suggests iron deficiency anaemia.

Eyes

Inspect the sclerae for jaundice, and the lower eyelid for anaemia.

Jaundice is easily overlooked. It is harder to detect in artificial lighting. Even the best examiner cannot detect bilirubin at 35 µmol/L, but everyone should notice a bilirubin over 50 µmol/L.

Face

Note abnormal pigmentation around the lips (e.g. in Peutz–Jeghers syndrome, which is rare except in examinations!) or angular stomatitis, which occurs in many medical conditions, especially iron deficiency anaemia, malabsorption, and oral infections.

Oral cavity

Inspect the oral cavity and tongue for:

- Ulceration (e.g. due to inflammatory bowel disease, chemotherapy, Behçet's syndrome).
- Inflammation.
- Oral candidiasis (e.g. secondary to antibiotic therapy, immunodeficiency, diabetes mellitus).
- Halitosis (e.g. due to infection, poor hygiene, hepatic foetor, uraemia, diabetes mellitus).

Chest wall

Note the presence of gynaecomastia and spider naevi. The presence of more than five spider naevi is considered to be suggestive of liver disease. These characteristically blanch if the central arteriole is pressed.

Supraclavicular lymphadenopathy

Pay particular attention to the left side and look for Virchow's node (Fig. 14.2). If present in a patient with intra-abdominal malignancy this is referred to as 'Troisers' sign'.

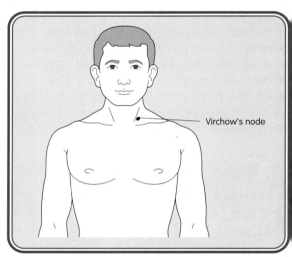

Virchow's node

Fig. 14.2 Virchow's node is a palpable left supraclavicular lymph node. Troisier's sign refers to the presence of a palpable left supraclavicular node in association with gastric carcinoma. This node is easiest to palpate from behind.

Exposure of the abdomen

Following general inspection, the abdomen should be exposed from the nipples to symphysis pubis. Follow the usual routine of inspection, palpation, percussion, and auscultation.

Inspection

Stand at the end of the bed and inspect the abdomen for:

- Symmetry (e.g. massive splenomegaly produces a bulge on the left side).
- Abnormal pulsation (e.g. due to abdominal aortic aneurysm).
- Shape (e.g. distension).

Examination Routine

Remember the six Fs as the causes of abdominal distension:
- Fat.
- Fluid.
- Faeces.
- Foetus.
- Fibroids.
- Flatus.

Return to the right-hand side of the patient and actively inspect for the presence of:
- Scars (Fig. 14.3).
- Sinuses (e.g. due to retained suture material).
- Fistulas (e.g. due to Crohn's disease).
- Visible peristalsis (e.g. due to intestinal obstruction).
- Distended veins.
- Flank haemorrhages (e.g. due to pancreatitis).

Ask patients whether they are aware of any abnormal lumps or areas of tenderness. This may give a clue to the area of pathology. Ask patients to cough, observing pain (peritoneal irritation) and also the hernial orifices.

Palpation

Before palpating, warn patients that you are going to lay your hand on their abdomen. It is courteous (and useful) to ask them to indicate any areas of tenderness or pain before palpation. The three stages to abdominal palpation are:
- Light palpation.
- Deep palpation.
- Specific palpation of the intra-abdominal organs.

Light palpation

Commence palpation at a site remote from the area of pain. All areas of the abdomen must be palpated systematically. Picture the abdomen in nine regions (Fig. 14.4). (Some people refer to abdominal quadrants as shown in Fig. 14.5.) This helps you to adopt a systematic approach to the examination and to the presentation of your findings.

Light palpation is performed to elicit any tenderness or guarding. Lay the hands and fingers

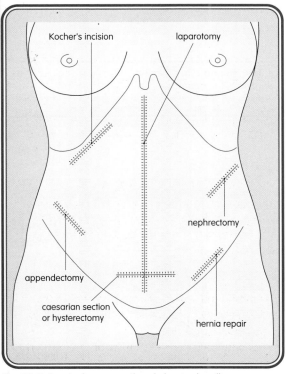

Fig. 14.3 Surgical scars on the abdominal wall.

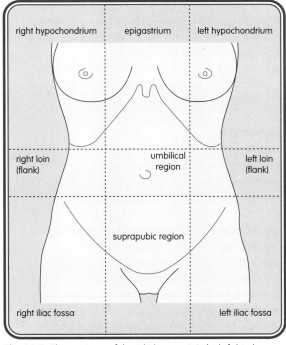

Fig. 14.4 The regions of the abdomen. It is helpful to be aware of these regions when palpating or presenting physical findings as this helps in the differential diagnosis.

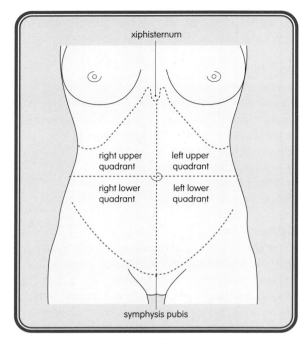

Fig. 14.5 The four quadrants of the abdomen.

flat upon the abdomen and press very gently. It may be necessary to kneel down beside the bed. It is essential to be as gentle as possible for two main reasons:

- To gain the patient's confidence.
- To prevent voluntary guarding (tensing of the abdominal wall musculature as light pressure is applied), which will mask pathological signs.

Deep palpation

Warn the patient that you will be pressing more firmly and feel for any obvious masses (Fig. 14.6) or tenderness in the nine regions. If a mass is identified, determine its characteristics systematically.

Specific palpation of the intra-abdominal organs

Liver: Always start in the right iliac fossa when examining the liver or the spleen as both expand towards this region. Place your hand flat with fingers pointing towards the patient's head (or alternatively to the left flank), and palpate deeply while asking the patient to breathe in and out deeply. Keep your hands still while the patient is breathing in as the liver edge moves downwards on inspiration. If nothing is felt, repeat the process with the hand slightly higher up the

abdomen, advancing a few centimetres at a time until the costal margin is reached.

The liver may be palpated in normal subjects, especially if they are thin or if there is chest hyperinflation (Fig. 14.7). If the liver edge is palpable, describe:

- The size of the liver.
- Its contour.
- Its texture.
- Any tenderness (see hepatomegaly, p. 120).

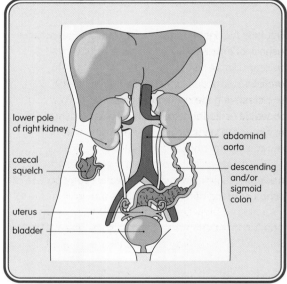

Fig. 14.6 Normal structures that may be palpable on deep palpation of the abdomen.

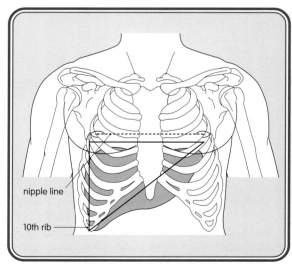

Fig. 14.7 Surface anatomy of the liver.

Spleen: The spleen is examined by a process similar to that for the liver. Start in the right iliac fossa with fingers pointing towards the left costal margin and ask the patient to breathe in and out while your fingers are advancing towards the left costal margin. If there is no obvious splenomegaly, ask the patient to roll onto the right side, place your left hand around the lower left costal margin and lift forwards as the patient inspires, while palpating with your right hand (Fig. 14.8).

A normal spleen is not palpable.

Kidneys: The kidneys are examined bimanually by the technique of ballottement. The left kidney is felt by placing your left hand in the left loin below the 12th rib lateral to the erector spinae muscles and above the iliac crest with the right hand placed anteriorly just above the anterior superior iliac spine. During inspiration, the left hand is then lifted upwards towards the right hand (Fig. 14.9).

The kidney may be palpable in thin normal individuals. The right kidney is examined with the right hand posteriorly and the left hand anteriorly.

In normal individuals, the right kidney lies lower than the left (due to downward displacement by the liver) and is more likely to be palpable (Fig. 14.10).

Abdominal aorta: Palpate specifically for an abdominal aortic aneurysm (AAA). This is performed by placing the palmar surfaces of both hands laterally and with the fingertips positioned in the midline a few centimetres below the xiphisternum (Fig. 14.11).

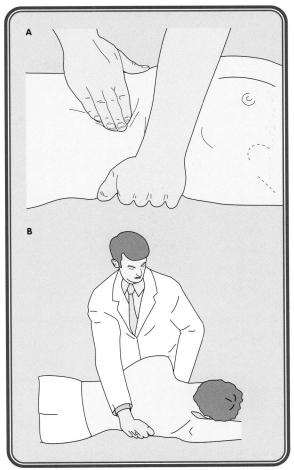

Fig. 14.8 Palpation of the spleen. (A) Initial examination. (B) If the examination is difficult, the patient should be asked to roll onto the right side; push the spleen forwards with your left hand and palpate with your right hand.

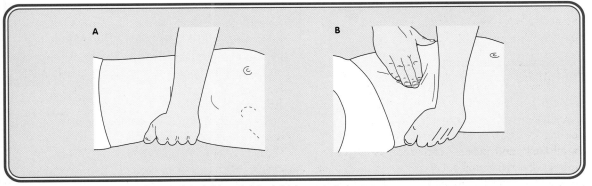

Fig. 14.9 Palpation of the kidneys. (A) Place left hand in the left loin posteriorly. (B) Place the right hand on the abdomen anteriorly and press gently downwards. Push the left hand upwards. A palpable kidney can be balloted between the two hands.

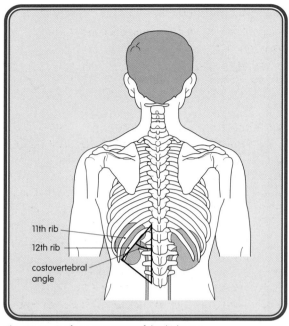

Fig. 14.10 Surface anatomy of the kidneys.

11th rib
12th rib
costovertebral angle

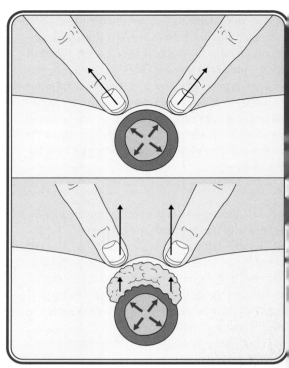

Fig. 14.12 Distinction between aortic pulsation and movement of an overlying structure. True pulsatility is indicated by outward displacement of the palpating hands.

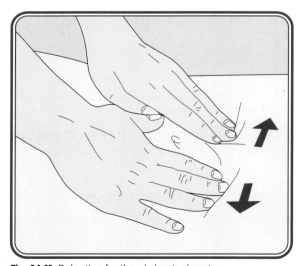

Fig. 14.11 Palpation for the abdominal aorta.

- An AAA is both pulsatile and expansile (fingertips will be pushed outwards).
- A non-aneurysmal abdominal aorta is only pulsatile (fingertips pushed upwards, but not outwards) (Fig. 14.12).

Percussion

Percuss over the whole abdomen and particularly over masses. This is also a sensitive method for eliciting peritonitis.

Specifically percuss for ascites by testing for shifting dullness. Percuss from the midline to the flank. If ascites is present, the initially resonant note will become dull. Note the point of transition on the skin, ask the patient to roll away from that side, wait a few seconds, and percuss over that area. If ascites is present the initially dull note will become resonant (Figs 14.13 and 14.14).

Auscultation

Listen specifically for bowel sounds. The presence or absence of bowel sounds is important. Listen for 30 seconds before concluding that bowel sounds are absent. Much mythology has been generated about the quality of these sounds, but this should be interpreted with caution. Listen specifically for bruits over the aorta and renal arteries.

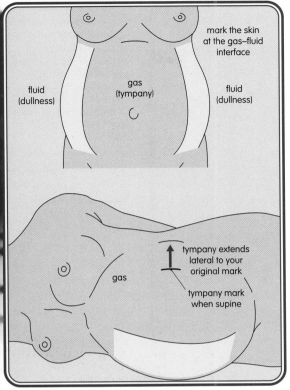

Fig. 14.13 Shifting dullness is a key sign of ascites. With the patient lying flat, percuss the abdomen sequentially from the umbilicus to the flank. Note the point at which the tympanic note becomes dull. Ask the patient to roll into the lateral position. Once the fluid has had time to move, the transition point from dullness to tympany will have altered.

Rectal examination

A complete abdominal examination includes assessment of:

- The hernial orifices.
- External genitalia.
- A rectal examination.

The rectal examination is usually performed with the patient in the left lateral position, with both hips and knees fully flexed (Fig. 14.15). It is essential to explain the procedure to the patient and to be gentle! Wear gloves and lubricate the finger. It is usually possible to palpate lesions up to 6–8 cm from the anal verge. Before performing a digital examination:

- Inspect the anus, its margins, and surrounding skin.
- Look for skin tags, excoriation, prolapsed or thrombosed haemorrhoids, fistulas, fissures, abscesses, or ulceration due to an anal carcinoma.
- Ask the patient to bear down or strain. This may reveal the presence of a rectal prolapse or occasionally a polyp.

While performing a digital rectal examination, the sphincter tone should be assessed and any tenderness elicited.

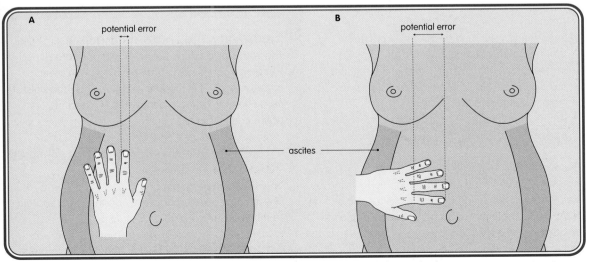

Fig. 14.14 Correct orientation of your hands is important when percussing the abdomen for the presence of ascites. (A) Correct positioning of the hand. (B) Incorrect positioning of the hand.

117

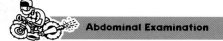
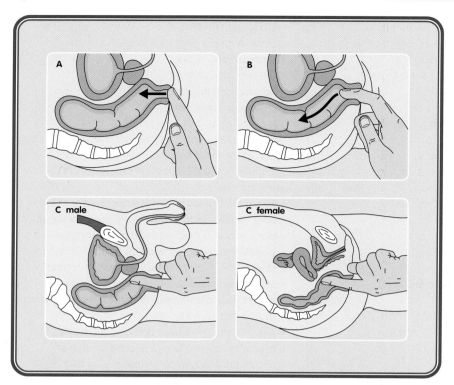

Fig. 14.15 The rectal examination. (A) Insert the tip of your index finger into the anal canal. (B) Follow the curve of the sacrum. (C) Sweep the finger around the pelvis, noting any irregularities, masses, or tenderness. Examine the glove on withdrawal of your finger.

Structures palpable during a normal digital rectal examination

Palpate anteriorly, laterally, and posteriorly. Note the following:

- Posteriorly—the tip of the coccyx and sacrum are palpable.
- Laterally—ischial spines and ischiorectal fossa.
- Anteriorly in males—prostate (smooth lateral lobes separated by the median sulcus); a prostatic carcinoma may be differentiated from benign prostatic hypertrophy by the loss of the median sulcus and possibly the presence of a palpable hard, craggy, irregular mass.
- Anteriorly in females—cervix through the vaginal wall and occasionally the body of the uterus.

The normal rectum may contain some faeces. Always look at the glove after examination for blood or mucus. Melaena stool has the appearance of sticky tar and an offensive characteristic smell. A rectal carcinoma may be palpable as a shelf-like lesion associated with blood on the glove.

Always wipe the patient after examination and offer further tissues.

Urinalysis

Urinalysis is particularly important in the context of abdominal pain (the urinary tract may be a source of pain), anaemia (haematuria) or jaundice (bilirubin).

HEPATOMEGALY

Identifying the mass as the liver

The liver is palpable in the right upper quadrant. Hepatomegaly is not usually confused with other organomegaly, but the liver should be distinguished from an enlarged right kidney. The features of hepatomegaly include:

- Palpable below the right costal margin (in gross hepatomegaly, it may extend to the left costal margin).
- Downward movement on inspiration.
- Dullness to percussion.
- It is impossible to palpate above the upper margin of the liver.

Characteristics of the liver

It is often possible to palpate a liver edge 1–2 cm below the right costal margin. If the liver edge is palpable, it is important to confirm that there is true hepatomegaly rather than a low diaphragm (e.g. due to chronic obstructive airways disease).

The size of the liver may be confirmed by percussion in a sagittal plane that records the 'height' of the liver. A normal liver is less than 15 cm. Record:

- Size of the liver. Once true hepatomegaly is confirmed, trace out the edge of the liver to define its margins. An enlarged right lobe (Riedel's lobe) is a normal finding. In the notes it is helpful to record accurately the size of the liver in the midclavicular line, midline, and if appropriate the left midclavicular line (Fig. 14.16).
- Consistency of the liver (e.g. hard, firm).
- Definition of the liver edge (e.g. smooth, knobbly).
- Tenderness (e.g. engorged liver in right heart failure).
- Pulsatility (e.g. as in tricuspid stenosis).

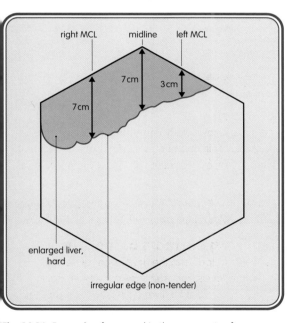

Fig. 14.16 Example of a record in the case notes for hepatomegaly. (MCL, mid-clavicular line.)

Aetiology

It is important to look for other features on systemic examination if hepatomegaly is found, as they may give clues to the underlying pathology (Fig. 14.17). In particular look for:

- Signs of chronic liver disease (e.g. due to alcoholic cirrhosis).

- Splenomegaly (e.g. due to portal hypertension, lymphoma).
- Generalized lymphadenopathy (e.g. due to lymphoma, carcinoma).
- Jugular venous wave (e.g. due to right heart failure, tricuspid regurgitation).
- Features of underlying malignancy.

Assessing severity

Look for features of hepatic decompensation, for example:

- Features of chronic liver disease (e.g. testicular atrophy, loss of axillary hair, gynaecomastia, spider naevi, leuconychia). These features suggest that the underlying disease process is chronic.
- Signs of portal hypertension. Always specifically check for ascites and splenomegaly. Look for a 'caput medusae' (dilated collateral veins radiating from the umbilicus).
- Signs of hepatic encephalopathy. Check the patient's mental state (especially for level of consciousness and constructional apraxia, Fig. 14.18.). Specifically check for a metabolic flap (asterixis) and foetor hepaticus.
- Jaundice.

SPLENOMEGALY

Identifying the mass as the spleen

A mass in the left upper quadrant is usually a spleen. It is not normal to be able to palpate the spleen. It must be enlarged 2 to 3-fold before it becomes palpable. It must be distinguished from the left kidney. The characteristics of the spleen on physical examination include:

- Presence in the left upper quadrant.
- Upper edge not palpable.
- Expansion towards the right lower quadrant.
- On inspiration, movement towards the right lower quadrant.
- A notch may be palpable.
- Dullness to percussion. The dullness extends above the costal margin.
- Not ballottable.

Assessing spleen size

Define the size of the spleen in a similar way to hepatomegaly (see p. 120). Note the descent of the

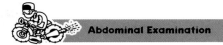

Fig. 14.17 Causes of hepatomegaly. * indicates the most common causes.

Causes of hepatomegaly	
Causes	**Features on examination**
cirrhosis*	features of chronic liver disease; features of portal hypertension; hard irregular, knobbly liver common
alcoholic	common; look for evidence of alcoholic toxicity in other systems (e.g. neuropathy)
primary biliary	usually middle-aged female; pruritus common (look for excoriation); xanthelasma
haemochromatosis	skin pigmentation; gonadal atrophy; more common in men
α-1-antitrypsin deficiency	signs of chronic obstructive airways disease
secondary carcinoma*	hard irregular knobbly liver edge; systemic features of malignancy (e.g. cachexia, etc.); lymphadenopathy; signs of primary malignancy (e.g. palpable breast lump, etc.)
congestive cardiac failure*	raised jugular venous pressure; peripheral oedema prominent; third heart sound; look for features of tricuspid regurgitation
infections (hepatitis A, B, C—rarely; glandular fever; cytomegalovirus; leptospirosis; hydatid; amoebic)	features are usually apparent from the history, but look for generalized lymphadenopathy
lymphoproliferative disorder (lymphoma; leukaemia; polycythaemia)	splenomegaly; generalized lymphadenopathy; anaemia or plethora; petechiae; etc.
miscellaneous amyloid polycystic fatty liver	splenomegaly; waxy skin; chronic disease palpable kidneys; signs of uraemia

spleen in the left midclavicular line and midline (Fig. 14.19).

Aetiology

The more common causes of splenomegaly are illustrated in Fig. 14.20. In particular, note the presence of:

- Hepatomegaly—portal hypertension, lymphoproliferative disorder.
- Generalized lymphadenopathy—lymphoproliferative disorder.
- Size of spleen—massive splenomegaly is usually due to chronic malaria, kala-azar, myelofibrosis, or chronic myeloid leukaemia (CML); a barely palpable spleen has a much wider differential diagnosis (see Fig. 14.20).

figure provided by doctor	attempt at copying by encephalopathic patient
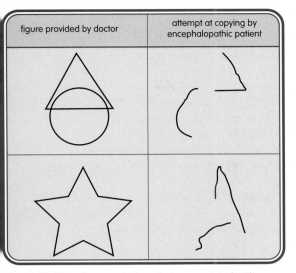

Fig. 14.18 Hepatic encephalopathy is associated with constructional apraxia. Ask the patient to copy a simple figure such as a five-pointed star or simple overlapping geometric shapes.

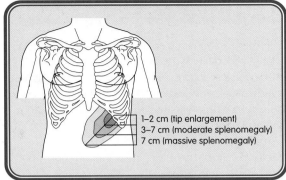

1–2 cm (tip enlargement)
3–7 cm (moderate splenomegaly)
7 cm (massive splenomegaly)

Fig. 14.19 Different degrees of splenomegaly.

Fig. 14.20 Causes of splenomegaly. The more important causes are marked with an asterisk. (CML, chronic myeloid leukaemia; SLE, systemic lupus erythematosus.)

Causes of splenomegaly	
Causes	**Features on examination**
lymphoproliferative disorders*	look for generalized lymphadenopathy and features of anaemia, thrombocytopenia, etc.
leukaemia*	massive in CML
lymphoma*	
polycythaemia rubra vera	plethora; hyperviscosity
myelofibrosis	usually massive
portal hypertension*	features of chronic liver disease; ascites; collateral veins on abdominal wall
(any cause of cirrhosis*, Budd–Chiari syndrome)	
infections*	
kala-azar, malaria (chronic)	massive splenomegaly; very important cause worldwide, but rarely seen in UK
glandular fever	widespread lymphadenopathy; usually young patient; look at throat
infective endocarditis	look for other stigmata and cardiac murmur (late sign)
miscellaneous	
amyloid	waxy skin; underlying disease; hepatomegaly
sarcoidosis	rash; arthropathy; Black patient, etc.
Felty's syndrome, SLE	arthritis, etc.
haemolytic anaemia	mild icterus; pallor

ANAEMIA

The causes of anaemia are widespread. The diagnosis is largely made from detailed laboratory testing and imaging investigations. However, it is essential that the investigation is focused and this relies upon a systematic assessment during the history (see p. 40) and examination.

Anaemia is usually detected clinically if the haemoglobin concentration is less than 10 g/dL . The signs of anaemia include:

- Conjunctival or mucosal pallor.
- Loss of colour in the palmar skin creases.

The more common causes of anaemia are:

- Iron-deficiency anaemia.
- Folate deficiency.
- Vitamin B_{12} deficiency.
- Haemolytic anaemia.

These diagnoses are insufficient, however, as an underlying cause still needs to be identified in order to provide suitable treatment and prognostic information.

Defining the cause of anaemia

A thorough systematic examination is essential. Clues may be found by considering the following.

General inspection

Inspect the face carefully. Look at the general health of the patient (e.g. cachexia suggests chronic disease), and note specifically any obvious disorders (e.g. rheumatoid arthritis). Some clues to iron deficiency and megaloblastic anaemia are illustrated in Fig. 14.21.

Note racial origin, for example:

- Mediterranean—thalassaemia.
- Afro-Caribbean—sickle cell anaemia.
- Northern European—hereditary spherocytosis.

Causes of blood loss

A systematic survey for a potential source of blood loss should be performed, for example:

- Abdominal scars.
- Gastrointestinal (GI) bleeding—look for abdominal masses; a rectal examination is mandatory.
- Genitourinary source—look for a palpable bladder or kidneys, perform urinalysis.

Features of chronic disease

Look for features of chronic disease such as:

- Infections (e.g. tuberculosis, osteomyelitis, infective endocarditis).
- Connective tissue disease.
- Crohn's disease.
- Malignancy.

Fig. 14.21 Features on general inspection of a patient with anaemia. * indicates the more common causes.

Features on general inspection in an anaemic	
Causes	**Features**
iron deficiency*	koilonychia (spoon-shaped nails); painless glossitis; angular stomatitis
hereditary haemorrhagic telangiectasia	visible telangiectasia on face and mouth
Peutz–Jeghers syndrome	pigmented macules around the lips and mouth
megaloblastic anaemia*	mild jaundice (lemon-yellow tinge) due to ineffective erythropoiesis; beefy red swollen tongue; angular stomatitis
pernicious anaemia	usually middle-aged or elderly female; look for features of other autoimmune disease (e.g. vitiligo)

Pregnancy

Pregnancy may be associated with folate and iron deficiency.

Abdominal examination

Pathology of the GI tract may cause anaemia, for example:

- GI bleeding, malabsorption (e.g. due to coeliac disease)—iron-deficiency anaemia.
- Gastrectomy, blind loop syndrome, Crohn's disease—anaemia due to folate or vitamin B_{12} deficiency.

In addition an intra-abdominal malignancy may be detected.

Organomegaly is associated with different types of anaemia:

- Liver disease is associated with macrocytic anaemia.
- Splenomegaly may be responsible for haemolytic anaemia.
- A large uterus may be due to pregnancy or be a cause of blood loss.
- Polycystic kidneys may be a cause of chronic renal failure and consequent anaemia.

Signs of haemolysis

Splenomegaly or mild jaundice may indicate that the underlying cause is haemolysis.

Assessing severity of anaemia

Try to make an assessment of the functional consequences of the anaemia. It is often hard to correlate the degree of pallor with the haemoglobin level. The functional impact of anaemia depends upon the underlying condition, the age and fitness of the patient, and the speed of onset. Look for signs of decompensation, for example:

- Hypotension—rapid blood loss may result in hypovolaemia and hypotension; postural blood pressure is the most sensitive indicator.
- Tachycardia—this develops early as a means of increasing oxygen delivery to the peripheral tissues in anaemia.
- Dyspnoea—note the exercise tolerance of a patient (e.g. short of breath at rest or on climbing onto the examination couch).
- Heart failure—especially in the elderly.

ACUTE GASTROINTESTINAL BLEED

Assessing the functional impact

The first priority is to perform adequate resuscitation before determining the cause of an acute GI bleed. It is important to recognize which patients are in danger of exsanguination. The process of assessment and emergency treatment should run in parallel. The initial examination should be aimed at assessing evidence of circulatory compromise.

General observations

The patient may appear grey and clammy and have cool peripheries. Profound hypovolaemia may result in confusion or obtundation. Respiration may be rapid and deep.

Pulse rate

Tachycardia is an early sign of hypovolaemia.

Blood pressure

Frequent assessments of blood pressure should be used to assess the adequacy of volume repletion. If the patient appears haemodynamically stable, postural blood pressure should be measured.

Jugular venous pressure

This will always be low in hypovolaemic patients. Often a central venous line is inserted to guide fluid replacement.

Site of bleeding

It is often clear that the bleeding is from the upper or lower GI tract. The vast majority of patients presenting with an acute GI bleed have a lesion at the level of the duodenum or above. Features to suggest an upper GI tract source of bleeding include:

- Haematemesis. Exclude haemoptysis or epistaxis with swallowing and subsequent vomiting of blood.
- Frank blood or 'coffee ground' material in the nasogastric (NG) aspirate.
- Absence of a bilious NG aspirate.
- Melaena. It is essential to perform a rectal examination. A melaena stool indicates bleeding proximal to the right colon and bleeding of usually more than 500 mL in the previous 24 hours. Test the stool for occult blood to avoid confusion with

bismuth or iron in the stool. Note that the presence of blood per rectum does not always indicate a lower GI bleed as a very brisk upper GI bleed (e.g. due to an aortoduodenal fistula) can result in apparently fresh blood per rectum.

Features of a lower GI bleed include the passage of bright red blood per rectum (haematochezia). This is not pathognomonic (see above), but in the presence of haematochezia, if the bleeding is from the upper GI tract, the patient will invariably be profoundly hypovolaemic.

Performing a detailed abdominal examination

A systematic abdominal system examination may provide further clues to the cause, for example:

- Abdominal masses (tumours, diverticular masses, AAA).
- Signs of liver disease. GI bleeding is common in liver failure, particularly of an alcoholic aetiology.
- Surgical scars. May indicate previous peptic ulcer disease, for example.
- Hereditary haemorrhagic telangiectasia. This is rare. Look for telangiectasia on the lips or fingers.
- Rectal examination findings. Note stool colour. This may indicate the location of the bleeding point as well as the speed of bleeding.

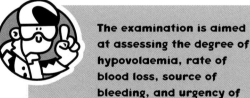

The examination is aimed at assessing the degree of hypovolaemia, rate of blood loss, source of bleeding, and urgency of resuscitation. The haemoglobin estimate in the first 24 hours may be misleading, so the requirement for blood transfusion relies upon thorough clinical assessment.

ACUTE ABDOMINAL PAIN

Acute abdominal pain is one of the most common causes of presentation to a casualty department. The differential diagnosis is vast, ranging from trivial conditions to life-threatening surgical emergencies. It is important to adopt a systematic approach to the examination. Consider the

differential diagnosis throughout the examination so that further management strategies can be instituted efficiently. The main aims of the examination are:

- To establish the cause of pain.
- To assess whether the patient would benefit from admission to hospital.
- To assess whether the patient requires surgical intervention.

General inspection

Before specifically examining the abdomen, look at the patient as a whole. It is helpful to ask the following questions.

Does the patient look unwell?

Patients with acute peritonitis usually look obviously unwell. They are disinterested in their surroundings and lie still so as not to aggravate the pain. Patients with renal colic may also appear distressed, but tend to be restless and in obvious pain. Conversely, patients who are laughing, smiling, or eating are most unlikely to have any significant acute surgical disease.

How old is the patient?

Different diseases are more common in different age groups. For example:

- Acute diverticulitis or AAA is much more common with increasing age.
- Acute appendicitis is commonest in young children and adolescents, but occurs in all age groups.
- Ectopic pregnancy will occur only in women of childbearing age.

What sex is the patient?

In women the differential diagnosis needs to be broadened to include gynaecological conditions. The other causes of intra-abdominal pain can occur in either sex, but some have a tendency to be more common in one sex. For example:

- Gallstones are more common in women.
- Peptic ulceration is more common in men.

Specific inspection

Perform a more specific inspection starting at the head and working down to the feet, noting the following.

General appearance

Cachexia may be due to chronic illness or malignancy.

Jaundice

The presence of jaundice should alert the doctor to:

- Gallstones—obstruction of the common bile duct, cholecystitis, pancreatitis.
- Chronic liver disease—associated with gastritis, acute alcoholic hepatitis, and pancreatitis as well as oesophageal varices.

Conjunctival pallor

In the context of acute abdominal pain, it may be hard to assess skin colouration as the patient often appears pale, grey, and sweaty. However, conjunctival pallor may suggest the presence of a chronic bleeding lesion, for example:

- Peptic ulcer.
- Colonic tumour with subsequent obstruction or intussusception.

Stigmata of chronic liver disease

See explanation of jaundice above.

Fever

The presence of fever suggests that an active inflammatory process is present.

Left supraclavicular lymphadenopathy

This is suggestive of intra-abdominal malignancy.

Checking vital signs

It is essential to check the vital signs as a baseline and to determine the urgency of therapy. Check the following.

Oral temperature

Even in the presence of peritonitis and active infection the patient may not have a fever, especially if shocked. However, the presence of pyrexia indicates that organic pathology is almost invariably present.

Pulse rate

It is unusual to have a tachycardia in the absence of active pathology. However, a very anxious patient may have tachycardia. The sequential recording of pulse rate is an accurate indicator of systemic disturbance if there is a progressive tachycardia (see Fig. 14.22). Rising pulse rate is also sometimes a more useful guide in elderly people whose temperature regulating mechanisms may be impaired.

Blood pressure

Check supine blood pressure. If the patient is able to cooperate, it is useful to check postural blood pressure. If the patient has shock or hypovolaemia there will be a drop in blood pressure on standing.

Fluid status

If the jugular venous waveform is easily visible, the jugular venous pressure provides a useful marker of fluid status.

Abdominal examination

Inspection

Inspect the abdomen noting:

- Visible peristalsis—suggestive of obstruction.
- Abdominal distension—may be due to obstruction.
- Rigidity—a tense, boardlike abdomen occurs in the presence of peritonitis.
- Any skin discolouration—pancreatitis may be associated with a bluish discolouration in the loins or umbilicus due to extravasation of bloodstained pancreatic juice into the retroperitoneum (Gray-Turner's and Cullen's signs).
- Obvious hernias.
- Abdominal scars—their presence raises the possibility of obstruction due to adhesions.
- Obvious organomegaly—for example massive polycystic kidneys may cause bulging in the flank. Bleeding into a cyst may be the cause of the pain.

Site of the pain

Ask the patient to show you exactly where the pain is on the abdomen. The location of the pain is the key to the underlying cause.

Examining the abdomen in detail

Perform a detailed abdominal examination as described at the start of this chapter. In particular, note:

- Presence or absence of signs of peritonitis.
- Presence of any abdominal masses.
- Location of the tenderness.

Signs of peritonitis

The presence of unexplained peritonitis is an indication for surgical intervention. The features of peritonitis are:

- Signs of shock (tachycardia, hypotension, which becomes progressive on serial observation; Fig. 14.22).
- Tenderness.
- Guarding (a sign of severe tenderness).

- Rebound tenderness. This is a useful discriminatory sign as many anxious patients have involuntary guarding upon palpation, but do not expect tenderness on withdrawal of the palpating hand. The tenderness may be distant to the site of palpation. Watch the patient's face for signs of rebound tenderness.
- Localized pain distant to the site of palpation.
- Absent bowel sounds.

Presence of an abdominal mass

Examination of palpable liver, spleen, and kidney is discussed on pp. 120, 121, and 132. In the context of acute abdominal pain, a mass in the right or left iliac fossa is most relevant.

Mass in the right iliac fossa

The most common causes are an appendix mass or carcinoma of the caecum. The differential diagnosis is shown in Fig. 14.23.

Mass in the left iliac fossa

The same diseases as those listed in Fig. 14.23 may cause a left iliac fossa mass, except carcinoma of the caecum, Crohn's disease, and tuberculosis. Diverticulitis is common and may cause a mass. Carcinoma of the colon usually presents with weight loss or a change in bowel habit, but occasionally presents as a left iliac fossa mass especially if it is causing obstruction.

Location of the pain

Generalized

Generalized abdominal pain is likely to be due to generalized peritonitis. The history is central to the diagnosis.

Epigastric

The most common causes of epigastric pain are:
- Peptic ulcer.
- A biliary cause (biliary colic or cholecystitis).
- Pancreatitis.

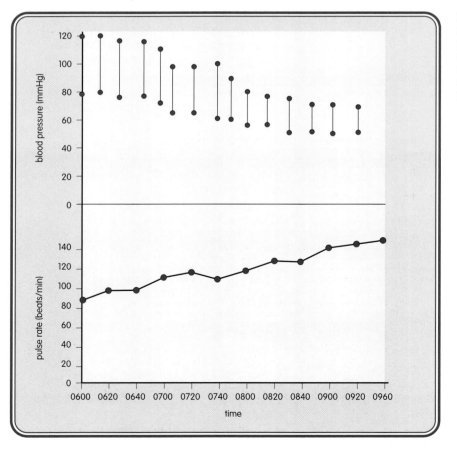

Fig. 14.22 The observation chart of a patient with peritonitis. Note the development of shock with a progressively rising pulse rate and decreasing blood pressure.

Peptic ulcer usually produces no signs unless perforation has occurred, though pyloric stenosis may result in visible peristalsis.

Biliary pain is more usually in the right upper quadrant. Often there are no abdominal signs, though there is commonly tenderness in the right upper quadrant upon inspiration.

Pancreatitis often produces surprisingly few abdominal signs for the degree of shock.

The conditions that cause abdominal pain, shock and a soft abdomen are:
- Pancreatitis.
- Bowel infarction.
- Dissection of an AAA.
- Referred pain from a myocardial infarction.

Loin pain
The main cause of loin pain are:
- Renal colic.
- Pyelonephritis.
- Musculoskeletal pain.

Right iliac fossa pain
The most important cause of right iliac fossa pain is acute appendicitis. However, the differential diagnosis is wide. Other causes include:
- Gastroenteritis.
- Mesenteric adenitis.
- Ruptured ovarian cyst.
- Acute salpingitis.
- Perforated peptic ulcer.
- Acute cholecystitis.
- Crohn's disease.
- Acute diverticulitis (rarely on the right).
- Renal colic.
- Ectopic pregnancy.

Medical conditions
It is important to remember that medical conditions may present with acute abdominal pain, so a detailed systemic examination is essential. In particular examine:
- The cardiovascular system. Inferior myocardial infarction or angina occasionally present with predominantly upper abdominal pain.
- The respiratory system. Pneumonia (especially with lower lobar disease) may cause right or left upper quadrant pain. Look for signs of consolidation.

Causes of a right iliac fossa mass	
Causes	**Features**
appendix mass	preceding history of central abdominal pain moving to the right iliac fossa; anorexia; tender mass; persistent fever and tachycardia; tender per rectum (PR)
carcinoma of the caecum	firm distinct mass; often non-mobile; usually non-tender; patient does not look acutely unwell
tuberculosis	more common in patients from the Indian subcontinent or Africa
Crohn's disease	patient may appear hypovolaemic owing to diarrhoea; oral aphthous ulcers; skin tags; mass usually mobile and of rubbery consistency; tender mass
psoas abscess	ill-defined mass; lumbar tenderness
iliac lymph nodes	
iliac artery aneurysm	

Fig. 14.23 Causes of a right iliac fossa mass.

15. Renal Examination

ACUTE RENAL FAILURE

If the cause of renal failure is not known, a thorough systemic examination is essential. Manifestations of the underlying diagnosis may be apparent from examination of any system.

Inspection

A detailed inspection is essential as many clues to the underlying cause of the renal failure may be manifest. Note:

- Any rash—for example livedo reticularis, vasculitic rash, cholesterol emboli, butterfly rash in systemic lupus erythematosus (SLE).
- Presence of oedema—nephrotic state versus intravascular fluid overload.
- General health—for example cachexia suggestive of malignancy.
- Jaundice—for example due to hepatorenal syndrome, leptospirosis.
- Pyrexia—for example due to infection, other inflammatory illness.
- Facial appearance—for example sunken nose in Wegener's granulomatosis.

Cardiovascular examination

Hypertension is common. It may be:

- The underlying cause of renal failure (look for retinopathy).
- The consequence, especially in the presence of fluid overload.

Assess fluid balance—note jugular venous pressure (JVP), oedema. Prerenal failure is the most common cause of renal failure in hospitalized patients. Listen for murmurs: mitral regurgitation is common in fluid overload; infective endocarditis can cause glomerulonephritis.

In addition, check peripheral pulses (renovascular disease is more likely if any peripheral pulse is absent or a bruit is audible).

Respiratory examination

Fibrosing alveolitis is associated with polyarteritis nodosa. Signs of consolidation may be due to infection or, in the context of renal failure, consider pulmonary haemorrhage.

Abdominal examination

A thorough abdominal examination is important, particularly certain features. For example:

- Palpable kidneys (e.g. polycystic kidneys, renal cell carcinoma).
- Epigastric bruits (suggesting renovascular disease).
- Abdominal masses (may be due to malignancy)— check for hepatomegaly, splenomegaly.
- Palpable bladder (e.g. due to obstructive uropathy).

Urinalysis is part of the clinical examination and is fundamental to the diagnosis of acute renal failure (see 'Abdominal examination', p. 120).

Neurological examination

Examine the fundi of all patients to reveal, for example, hypertension, diabetes mellitus, vasculitis. Mononeuritis multiplex (e.g. due to systemic vasculitis, SLE) is often associated with vasculitic illnesses.

Locomotor examination

Assess the presence of any active synovitis (e.g. SLE, rheumatoid arthritis). Rheumatoid arthritis may be associated with renal failure in a number of ways, for example due to:

- Vasculitis.
- Second-line drugs causing glomerulonephritis.
- Interstitial nephritis due to use of non-steroidal anti-inflammatory drugs (NSAIDs).
- Amyloid deposition as a consequence of the chronic inflammatory process.

Look for gouty tophi (urate nephropathy). In addition, the presence of a chronic arthralgia may be associated with analgesic nephropathy.

CHRONIC RENAL FAILURE

Patients with chronic renal failure often have specific problems, which should always be considered during an assessment. For dialysis patients, consider the following points.

Dialysis access
Haemodialysis
Note the presence of the arteriovenous fistula (AVF), its site (e.g. radial, brachial), and the palpable thrill. Look for access sites used and other possible access sites including Gortex graft, shunts, or central venous (polytetrafluoroethylene) catheters.

Look specifically for signs of infection (especially with venous catheters).

Peritoneal dialysis
Look at the exit site of the peritoneal dialysis catheter for evidence of tunnel infection or exit site infection. If the patient has reported abdominal symptoms, it is important to inspect the dialysis fluid for turbidity, blood, or cloudiness suggestive of peritonitis.

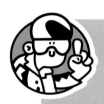

Measure the patient's weight at every visit. This is the most sensitive guide to changes in fluid balance on a day to day basis.

Assessing fluid balance
Fluid overload is a common problem in anuric patients.

Look for other signs of fluid overload such as:
- Raised JVP.
- Peripheral oedema—if the patient has a normal plasma albumin, peripheral oedema usually indicates a fluid overload of approximately 3 kg.
- Uncontrolled hypertension.
- Pulmonary oedema—often a combination of fluid overload and cardiac failure.

Some patients develop symptoms such as lightheadedness, fainting, or malaise towards the end of dialysis. Look for signs of dehydration such as:
- Dry mucous membranes.
- Postural hypotension.

Lying and standing blood pressure
Most dialysis patients have hypertension and strict blood pressure control is central to reducing long-term morbidity from cardiac disease. Postural blood pressure assessment is useful for determining fluid balance.

Erythropoietin therapy may exacerbate hypertension.

Activity of underlying disease
It is important to remember the underlying cause of renal failure as this may cause special problems in management. For example:
- The diabetic patient has a particularly high risk of cardiovascular disease.
- A patient with a vasculitic illness may develop recurrent vasculitis with extrarenal complications (e.g. pulmonary haemorrhage).
- Amyloid may progress, causing systemic complications.

Performing a full systemic examination
Renal failure is a multisystem disease, and a full assessment is essential.

Do not forget the original disease causing the renal failure!

PALPABLE KIDNEYS

It is unusual to be able to palpate the kidneys in any but the very lean patients. If a kidney is palpable, it is necessary to:
- Identify the mass as a kidney.
- Consider the underlying cause.

Identifying the mass as a kidney

A palpable kidney is rarely confused with any other organ, but it should be clearly differentiated from the spleen on the left and the liver on the right (Fig. 15.1).

The right kidney is often palpable in a thin subject; the left is palpable less often. Features of an enlarged palpable kidney include:

- Location in the loin (paracolic gutter).
- It is usually possible to palpate only the lower pole.
- Downward movement on inspiration (the spleen tends to move towards the right iliac fossa).
- Usually resonant to percussion (see spleen or liver, p. 120) as it is overlaid by the colon.
- It can be balloted (almost a pathognomonic sign).
- It may be possible to 'get above' the mass (compare directly with the liver or spleen, p. 120).

Characteristics of the kidney

Once the organ has been identified as a kidney, define the size, consistency, and shape. Listen over the organ for a bruit, which may be present if there is renal artery stenosis or a tumour.

Aetiology
Bilateral palpable kidneys

The most common causes of bilaterally palpable kidneys are:

- Polycystic kidneys (the most common cause). The kidneys may be massive. Most other causes of enlarged kidneys result in smooth hemi-ovoid masses, but occasionally individual cysts may be palpable. Look for an associated polycystic liver, signs of uraemia, or an arteriovenous fistula.
- Bilateral hydronephrosis.
- Amyloidosis. The patient may have a typical facies, hepatosplenomegaly, peripheral neuropathy, or obvious underlying inflammatory disease (e.g. rheumatoid arthritis, chronic osteomyelitis).

Do not forget to check the urinalysis.

Other causes are shown in Fig. 15.2.

Unilateral palpable kidney

The most common causes are similar to those of bilateral palpable kidneys, but in order of frequency include:

- Polycystic kidneys.
- Renal cell carcinoma.
- Hydronephrosis.
- Hypertrophy of a single functioning kidney (kidney only just palpable).

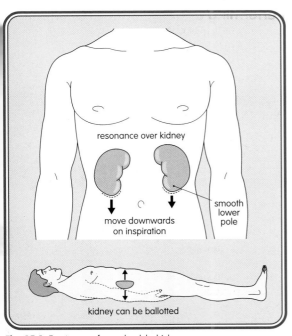

resonance over kidney

move downwards
on inspiration

smooth
lower
pole

kidney can be balloted

Fig. 15.1 Features of a palpable kidney.

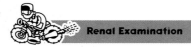

Causes of single or bilaterally enlarged kidneys	
Causes	**Features**
polycystic kidneys	usually bilateral; large cysts may be individually detected; check blood pressure; note uraemic complications; may detect hepatomegaly
hydronephrosis	unilateral or bilateral; may be tender if acute; check prostate and palpable bladder
malignancy Wilms' tumour (child) renal cell carcinoma (hypernephroma)	look for systemic features of malignancy
miscellaneous pyonephrosis single cyst amyloid	 tender usually incidental finding rare; look for underlying disease

Fig. 15.2 Causes of single or bilaterally enlarged kidneys.

16. Neurological Examination

EXAMINATION ROUTINE

The neurological examination is often considered by students to be the most difficult part of the examination and is most commonly omitted. In a routine assessment, it is essential to perform at least a basic neurological assessment. This need not take more than a few minutes, but provides essential information.

More than in any other system, it is vital to be systematic, objective, and methodical, and to be aware of the pathological significance of any elicited sign. It is essential to record exactly what has been assessed rather than meaningless phrases (e.g. 'CNS—tick'). Interpretation of neurological conditions often relies on changes of neurological signs with time, highlighting the need to ensure accuracy when writing up the medical record.

Cranial nerves

It is important to understand the basic anatomy and function of the individual cranial nerves when interpreting physical findings. For each cranial nerve, function, anatomy, examination routine, and interpretation of the physical signs will be considered.

Olfactory nerve (cranial nerve I)
Function
The olfactory nerve is a sensory nerve conveying the sense of smell.

Anatomy
Nerve fibres pass from sensory receptors in the nasal cavity through the cribriform plate to the olfactory bulb, where they synapse, and then pass towards the anterior perforated substance.

Examination
Ask patients whether they have noticed any change in their sense of smell. Test smell in each nostril separately using a sniff test. Use common, easily recognizable, non-irritant substances (e.g. vanilla, orange, coffee).

Interpretation
It is relatively unusual to detect lesions of the olfactory nerve on physical examination. Formal testing is rarely needed unless a lesion of the anterior cranial fossa is suspected. If a lesion is detected, note the following:
- Anosmia is usually due to nasal rather than neurological disease.
- The olfactory nerve is vulnerable as it passes through the cribriform plate, especially if there is a head injury. Also consider frontal lobe tumours and meningitis (infective or neoplastic).

Optic nerve (cranial nerve II)
Function
The optic nerve is a sensory nerve conveying the sense of vision from the retina.

Anatomy
The optic nerve leaves the eye via the optic foramen, partially decussates at the optic chiasm, and synapses at the lateral geniculate nucleus. Secondary fibres pass to the occipital cortex via the optic radiation (see 'Interpretation' below).

Examination
Visual acuity: Assess distant and near vision formally using Snellen and Jaeger charts allowing patients to wear their spectacles, or crudely at the bedside (e.g. count fingers from two metres or read newsprint) for each eye (see p. 189, and Fig. 21.1).

Visual fields: Test by confrontation. Sit opposite the patient approximately one metre away at the same level. Both patient and examiner cover one eye, and the examiner brings a test object (traditionally a white hatpin, but in the clinic other objects may need to be substituted, e.g. a pen top) into the field of vision from each quadrant midway between himself and the patient. The patient states when he or she first sees the object, and the examiner can then compare the patient's visual field directly with his own.

Pupillary reflexes: These are discussed under oculomotor nerve (see p. 137).

Fundoscopy: See Chapter 23, p. 190 for detail.

Interpretation

Visual field defects should be correlated with the anatomical site of the lesion. It is helpful to understand the visual pathway (Fig. 16.1).

Oculomotor, trochlear, and abducens nerves (cranial nerves III, IV, VI)

Function

The oculomotor, trochlear, and abducens nerves are considered together as they supply the extraocular muscles (Fig. 16.2). The oculomotor nerve also supplies levator palpebrae superioris, which opens the upper eyelid. In addition, it also has parasympathetic fibres supplying the sphincter pupillae (constricts the pupil) and the ciliary muscle of lens.

Anatomy

The oculomotor nucleus lies in the midbrain. It passes close to the posterior communicating artery before entering the lateral wall of the cavernous sinus on the way to the orbit.

The trochlear nucleus lies lower in the midbrain. Fibres pass dorsally, decussate, pass around the midbrain, and enter the lateral wall of the cavernous sinus.

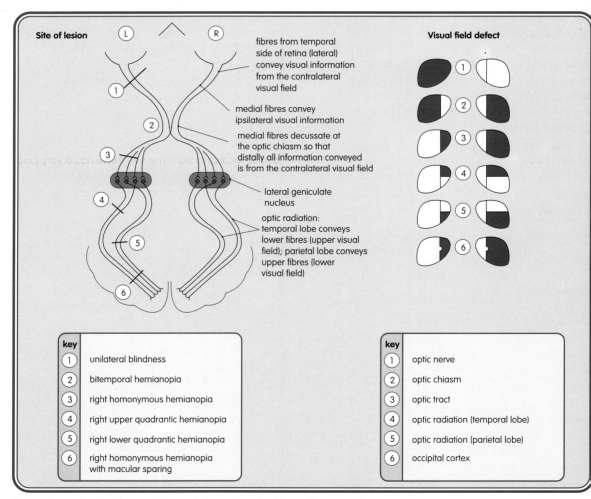

Fig. 16.1 The visual pathway. Lesions at different parts of the pathway produce characteristic field defects.

Nerve supply and movement produced by the extraocular muscles		
Nerve	**Muscle**	**Movement**
oculomotor	medial rectus	adduction
	inferior rectus	inferior movement (especially when eye abducted)
	superior rectus	superior movement
	inferior oblique	superior movement (especially when eye adducted)
trochlear	superior oblique	inferior movement (especially when eye adducted)
abducens	lateral rectus	abduction

Fig. 16.2 Nerve supply and movement produced by the extraocular muscles.

The abducens nerve originates close to the facial nerve in the pons, emerges in the cerebellopontine angle and has a very long intracranial course, passing over the petrous temporal bone on the way to the cavernous sinus.

Examination

Inspection: Look at the eyelids for ptosis and symmetry.

Pupils: Look at pupil size and symmetry. Test the pupillary reflex by shining light on the pupil from the side, looking at both the direct and the consensual response.

Ocular movements: Observe the patient following a target up, down, to either side, and for convergence. Note diplopia or nystagmus.

Interpretation

When interpreting physical signs, note the following:
- Ptosis (Fig. 16.3).
- Abnormal pupillary reflexes. The afferent limb is from the optic nerve, the efferent pathway is via the oculomotor nerve. An intact consensual reflex with an absent direct reflex implies a lesion of the IIIrd nerve. Conversely, pupil constriction only when light is shone into the opposite eye implies a sensory deficit.
- Holmes–Adie pupil. This is common in normal women. The pupil is large with an absent light reflex and delayed accommodation reflex, which is sustained. It is often associated with absent ankle reflexes.
- Nystagmus. This may be due to visual disturbances or lesions of the labyrinth, cerebellum, brainstem, or central vestibular connections.
- VIth nerve palsy (loss of eye abduction). This is often a false localizing sign. The VIth nerve has a very long intracranial course and is vulnerable to compression

Fig. 16.3 Causes of ptosis. (CVA, cerebrovascular accident)

Causes of ptosis	
Cause	**Examples**
third nerve palsy complete ptosis, associated with widely dilated pupil, and eye paralysed with outward and downward deviation	posterior communicating artery aneurysm 'coning' of the temporal lobe mononeuritis multiplex (e.g. due to diabetes mellitus, vasculitis) midbrain lesion
Horner's syndrome loss of sympathetic supply to eye, partial ptosis, pupillary constriction, enophthalmos and decreased sweating on affected side	brain lesions (e.g. CVA lateral medullary syndrome) cervical cord lesions (e.g. syringomyelia) T1 root lesion (e.g. apical lung cancer, cervical rib) sympathetic chain lesion (e.g. neoplasia)
neuromuscular disease	myasthenia gravis botulism
myogenic	senile degenerative changes dystrophia myotonica

as it passes over the petrous temporal bone. Any pathology causing raised intracranial pressure may result in a VIth nerve palsy.

- VIth nerve lesions may be due to a lesion in the pons or cerebellopontine angle. This often occurs in association with a VIIth (or VIIIth) nerve palsy and may result in contralateral pyramidal tract signs.

- IVth nerve palsy. This rarely occurs in isolation. Orbital trauma often damages the tendon, causing muscular weakness.

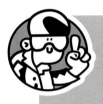

Sixth nerve palsy is commonly a false localizing sign and results from raised intracranial pressure.

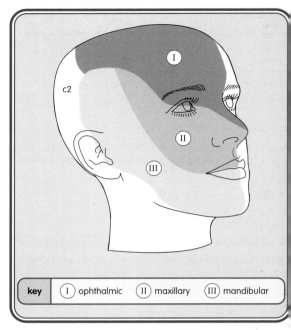

| key | (I) ophthalmic | (II) maxillary | (III) mandibular |

Fig. 16.4 Dermatomes of the three divisions of the trigeminal nerve.

Trigeminal nerve (cranial nerve V)

Function

The trigeminal nerve conveys sensory and motor nerve fibres. The main functions are:

- Sensory—somatic sensation to the face.
- Motor—muscles of mastication (masseters, temporalis, pterygoids).

Anatomy

The trigeminal nerve is split into the following three divisions (Fig. 16.4):

- Ophthalmic.
- Maxillary.
- Mandibular.

The trigeminal ganglion lies near the pons. The nerve fibres pass near the medial lemniscus to the thalamus.

Examination

Sensory: Test modalities of sensation over the three distributions of the nerve (e.g. forehead, cheeks, chin) bilaterally.

Corneal reflex: Lightly touch the cornea with cotton wool, approaching from the side, and observe a brisk contraction of orbicularis oris (blinking).

Motor: Inspect for wasting of the temporalis and masseter muscles. Test jaw opening against resistance (unilateral pterygoid weakness will cause the jaw to deviate to the side of the weakness).

Jaw jerk: With the mouth slightly open and the jaw relaxed, place your index finger over the mandible and gently strike it with a tendon hammer. Look for reflex closing of the mouth. This is often difficult to interpret as it is frequently absent.

Interpretation

When examining the Vth nerve, note the following points:

- An absent corneal reflex may be the first sign of ophthalmic herpes zoster. Lesions of the Vth and VIIth nerves can be distinguished by comparing the contralateral responses. The afferent limb is from the Vth nerve, the efferent limb is provided by the facial nerve, and is usually bilateral.

- Central lesions are often associated with other localizing signs (e.g. first division in association with IIIrd, IVth and VIth nerve lesions in the cavernous sinus; cerebellopontine angle lesions).
- Sensory lesions are much more common than motor lesions.

Facial nerve (cranial nerve VII)
Function
The facial nerve is primarily a motor nerve, but conveys fibres of three different modalities:
- Motor—to muscles of facial expression.
- Parasympathetic—to lacrimal, submaxillary, and sublingual glands.
- Sensory—taste for the anterior two-thirds of the tongue and an insignificant part of the external ear.

Anatomy
The motor nucleus lies in the pons close to the VIth nerve. It emerges in the cerebellopontine angle and enters the internal auditory meatus with the VIIIth nerve, giving off the nerve to stapedius and chorda tympani (taste) before emerging through the stylomastoid foramen and passing peripherally through the parotid gland, giving off various branches.

Examination
Inspection: Inspect the face for:
- Asymmetry (e.g. loss of nasolabial fold, drooping and dribbling from corner of mouth, weak smile).

- Facial expression.
- Involuntary movements.

Muscle strength: Examine the individual muscles. The lower face may be assessed by smiling, whistling, pursing lips; the upper face by closure of eyes, elevation of eyebrows, frowning.

Taste: Taste is rarely formally tested.

Interpretation
By far the most important component of the facial nerve is motor. Upper motor neuron (UMN) lesions often result in relative preservation of movements of the upper face due to crossed innervation (Fig. 16.5). In addition, emotional expression may be preserved. Lower motor neuron (LMN) VIIth nerve lesions do not spare the muscles around the eyes. The site of the lesion can often be localized, for example to the:
- Pons—for example due to a cerebrovascular accident (CVA); associated with VIth nerve lesion and contralateral pyramidal tract signs.
- Cerebellopontine angle—for example due to an acoustic neuroma; associated with lesions of the VIth and VIIIth nerves as well as cerebellar ataxia.
- Facial canal—for example due to Bell's palsy, herpes zoster; associated with loss of taste and hyperacusis as well as weakness of the muscles of facial expression.
- Parotid gland—for example due to sarcoidosis, parotid tumour; individual facial muscles may be affected.

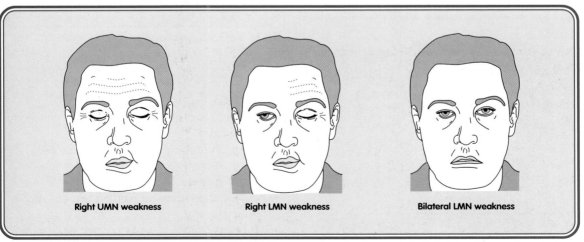

Fig. 16.5 Facial weakness. Patients are asked to close their eyes and purse their lips. Note the failed eye closure in lower motor neuron (LMN) lesions and the nasolabial fold with drooping mouth in both upper motor neuron (UMN) and LMN lesions.

Vestibulocochlear nerve (cranial nerve VIII)

Function

The vestibulocochlear nerve is a sensory nerve. It has two primary functions:

- Auditory—sense of hearing.
- Labyrinthine—sense of balance.

Anatomy

Auditory: Sensory fibres from the cochlea enter the cerebellopontine angle in association with the facial nerve, synapse in the lower pons, and ascend in the lateral lemnisci.

Vestibular: Fibres pass with the auditory division, but synapse in the vestibular nucleus in the medulla, from which there are connections to the cerebellum, extraocular muscles, and higher centres.

Examination

Auditory: Crude assessment can be made for each ear (e.g. "can hear whispered voice"). If a defect is found, conductive or sensory deficits may be identified using tuning fork tests (Fig. 16.6) as follows:

- Rinne's test—using a 256 Hz tuning fork, compare subjective loudness when it is presented close to the external auditory meatus and when the base is applied to the mastoid—a positive test (normal) occurs if the former appears louder.
- Weber's test—apply the base of the tuning fork to the middle of the forehead and ask the patient whether he or she hears the sound in the midline or to one side—the test is abnormal if the sound is lateralized.

Vestibular: This function is not routinely tested. Positional nystagmus can be observed by holding the patient's head over the end of the examination couch and then fully extending and turning it with the eyes open. This test is called Hallpike's manoeuvre (Fig. 16.7).

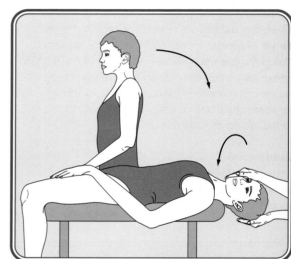

Fig. 16.7 Hallpike's manoeuvre for testing positional nystagmus.

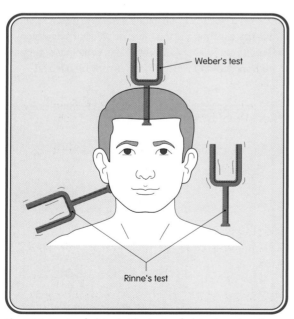

Fig. 16.6 Tuning fork tests. The tuning fork is placed on the vertex of the head in Weber's test. In Rinne's test a tuning fork is struck and placed close to the external ear and rested on the mastoid process to test air and bone conduction.

Interpretation

If hearing loss is identified, try to identify the underlying cause. Note that:

- Tuning fork tests are useful for identifying the hearing deficit as primarily conductive or sensory in origin (Fig. 16.8).
- Deafness is commonly conductive (e.g. due to otitis media, ear wax).
- Sensory deafness can be further defined by formal audiometry to quantify and define the frequency range of hearing loss.

Assessment of tuning fork tests			
Condition	Rinne's (left ear)	Rinne's (right ear)	Weber's
normal hearing	positive	positive	heard in midline
conductive deficit in right ear	positive	negative	heard on right side
sensory deficit in right ear	positive	positive	heard on left side

Fig. 16.8 Assessment of tuning fork tests.

Vertigo is most commonly peripheral. Central lesions (e.g. cerebellar lesions) are not associated with deafness or tinnitus, but are often associated with pronounced ataxia between the episodes of vertigo and persistent nystagmus.

Glossopharyngeal nerve (cranial nerve IX)
Function
The glossopharyngeal nerve has three functions:
- Sensory—taste for the posterior one third tongue, most of oropharynx, and soft palate.
- Parasympathetic (parotid gland).
- Motor—to stylopharyngeus.

Anatomy
The motor and sensory nuclei lie in the medulla. The nerve leaves the skull with the Xth and XIth nerves at the jugular foramen.

Examination
Gag reflex: Ask the patient to say "aah" with his or her mouth open and observe palatal movement. Touch the posterior wall of the oropharynx with an orange stick on each side. This elicits constriction and elevation. If there is no response, ask the patient whether he or she felt the stimulus.

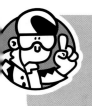

The gag reflex is unpleasant, and should be performed only if a lesion of the IXth or Xth nerves is suspected.

Interpretation
The afferent limb of the gag reflex is via the IXth nerve, the efferent from the Xth.

Vagus nerve (cranial nerve X)
Function
The vagus nerve supplies innervation to the viscera in the thorax and foregut as well as having smaller motor and sensory functions. The main functions are:
- Parasympathetic—visceral innervation to heart, lungs, foregut.
- Motor—to larynx, soft palate, pharynx.
- Sensory—for dura mater of the posterior cranial fossa, small part of the external ear.

Anatomy
The nucleus lies in the medulla.

Examination
Speech: Listen for dysphonia or a bovine cough associated with recurrent laryngeal nerve palsy.

Soft palate: Observe the uvula. In a unilateral lesion, it will droop away from the lesion.

Gag reflex: See above for glossopharyngeal nerve.

Interpretation
In the presence of dysphonia, the vocal cords should be examined.

Accessory (spinal accessory) nerve (cranial nerve XI)
Function
The spinal accessory nerve is a motor nerve supplying the sternomastoid and trapezius muscles.

139

Anatomy

The anterior horn cells of the cervical cord innervate these muscles, but fibres pass up to the medulla before descending again through the jugular foramen.

Examination

Test the bulk and power of sternomastoid. Ask patients to:

- Force their chin downwards against the resistance of your hand (this tests the power of the sternomastoid muscle bilaterally).
- Turn chin to one side against resistance (unilateral weakness affects turning to the opposite side).

The power of trapezius can be tested by asking patients to shrug their shoulders against resistance.

Hypoglossal nerve (cranial nerve XII)

Function

The hypoglossal nerve is a motor nerve supplying innervation to the muscles of the tongue.

Anatomy

The nucleus is in the medulla.

Examination

Inspection: Look at the tongue for wasting and fasciculation.

Protrusion: Ask patients to protrude their tongue. If there is a unilateral lesion, the tongue will deviate towards the side of the lesion.

Motor system

When examining the motor system, the aim is to:

- Identify any lesions.
- Ascertain whether the lesion is an UMN or LMN lesion.
- Locate the anatomical site of the lesion.
- Consider the differential diagnosis of lesions at that site.

The fundamental distinction is between UMN (above the anterior horn cells) and LMN lesions (Fig. 16.9).

The examination should follow a strict routine of:

- Inspection.
- Palpation.
- Assessment of muscular tone.
- Assessment of power.
- Assessment of tendon reflexes.
- Assessment of coordination.
- Assessment of gait.

Inspection

Inspection should begin as the patient enters the examination room. Observe the patient as he or she approaches you. Obvious abnormalities in posture, gait, co-ordination or involuntary movements should be noted. The patient should be fully exposed in his or her underwear on the examination couch so that individual muscle groups can be observed. Inspect specifically for:

- Wasting—note symmetry; look specifically for distribution (e.g. proximal wasting).
- Fasciculation (spontaneous contraction of small groups of muscle fibres)—usually implies a LMN lesion (e.g. motor neuron disease).
- Tremors—note whether coarse or fine and whether a resting tremor or an intention tremor.

Features of UMN and LMN lesions	
UMN	**LMN**
no muscle wasting (but there may be disuse atrophy)	wasting
increased tone ('clasp-knife')	flaccid
weakness of characteristic distribution	marked weakness
hyperreflexia	depressed or absent reflex
abnormal plantar response	normal plantar response
no fasciculation	fasciculation

Fig. 16.9 Features of upper motor neuron (UMN) and lower motor neuron (LMN) lesions.

Palpation

Palpate the muscle groups, specifically noting:
- Muscle bulk.
- Tenderness (e.g. myositis).

Assessment of muscular tone

Normally, there is a limited resistance through the range of movement.

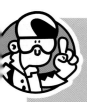

When assessing muscular tone it is essential that the patient is properly relaxed and lying in a neutral position.

If increased tone is suspected, attempt to elicit clonus (Fig. 16.10). Assessment of tone is subjective and requires experience, but specifically consider:
- Hypertonia—for example 'clasp-knife' (high resistance to initial movement and then sudden release; characteristic of UMN lesions), 'lead-pipe rigidity' (resistance through the range of movement; in

Parkinson's disease this in combination with the tremor produces 'cogwheel rigidity').
- Hypotonia—for example due to LMN and cerebellar lesions.

Assessment of power

Individual muscle groups should be tested to assess power. When testing, patients should be at a slight mechanical advantage so that if they have normal power, they can just overcome the resistance of the examiner. Muscle strength should be classified according to the Medical Research Council (MRC) grade (Fig. 16.11).

It is usually sufficient to test:
- Movements of the neck.
- Shoulder abduction and adduction.
- Movements of the elbows, wrists, and hands.
- Movements of the hips, knees, and ankle.

When detecting a weakness, it should be categorized as either UMN or LMN. If classified as LMN, the physical signs should be integrated to identify the lesion anatomically (Fig. 16.12).

When testing each muscle group, always consider:
- The myotome.
- The peripheral nerve supplying the muscles.

Fig. 16.10 Technique of eliciting ankle clonus. Bend the patient's knee slightly, supporting it with one hand. Grasp the forefoot with the other hand and suddenly dorsiflex the foot. Clonus is made up of regular oscillations of the foot. Sustained (> 4 beats) clonus indicates an upper motor neuron (UMN) lesion. One or two beats is normal.

MRC classification of muscle power	
Grade	**MRC grade of muscle strength**
0	no movement
1	flicker of movement visible
2	movement possible with gravity eliminated
3	movement possible against gravity, but not resistance
4	movement possible against resistance, but weakened (often subdivided to 4−, 4, 4+)
5	normal power

Fig. 16.11 Medical Research Council (MRC) classification of muscle power.

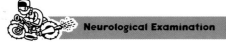

Location of lesion	Examples	Features
anterior horn cells	motor neuron disease; polio	usually symmetrical; no myotome/ nerve root distribution; often distal initially; no sensory involvement
nerve root (radiculopathy)	nerve root compression	distribution of affected muscles according to myotome; may have associated dermatomal sensory loss
peripheral nerve (neuropathy)	carpal tunnel	weakness according to nerve supply of affected nerve; usually associated sensory loss; early loss of reflexes
neuromuscular junction	myasthenia gravis	loss of power fluctuating in severity, not in distribution of peripheral nerve or myotome
muscle (myopathy)	n.a.	often has characteristic distribution of a particular disease; reflexes may be preserved early in disease; no sensory loss

Features of LMN lesions originating in the spinal cord, nerve root, peripheral nerve, neuromuscular junction, and muscle

Fig. 16.12 It is usually possible to localize a lower motor neuron (LMN) lesion as originating in the spinal cord, nerve root, peripheral nerve, neuromuscular junction, or muscle.

The major movements in the upper and lower limbs are illustrated in Figs 16.13, 16.14, and 20.4. It is essential to be systematic if a weakness is identified, so that the pattern of involvement can be recognized as corresponding to a nerve root, peripheral nerve, or an individual muscle group (Fig. 16.15). This can be correlated with the other features of the examination of the peripheral nervous system.

Specific tests for the more common peripheral neuropathies are considered below on p. 152.

Assessment of tendon reflexes

The reflexes should be elicited using a tendon hammer. Compare the relative responses, both against normality and with each side. Make a note of the response— whether it appears normal, brisk, or reduced. If no response is obtained, try methods to reinforce the reflex. For example ask patients to clench their teeth or hook their fingers around each other and try to separate their hands without disentangling their fingers (Fig. 16.16). The nerve roots of the more commonly elicited reflexes are listed in Fig. 16.17 and the reflex arc is shown in Fig. 16.18.

Disruption of the reflex may be due to a lesion at the level of the:

- Peripheral nerves (peripheral neuropathy). Typically the reflex is depressed early in the course of the pathology.
- Spinal cord.
- Neuromuscular junction.
- Muscle (myopathy). The reflex is usually retained until late in the natural history of the disease.

Assessment of coordination

Coordination in the upper limb is tested by the finger–nose test. Hold a finger at arm's length from patients and then ask them to touch the tip of their nose rapidly, and then the tip of your finger with their index finger. The smoothness and accuracy of the movements should be interpreted and put into context with any muscle weakness.

The lower limbs may be assessed by the heel–shin test. Ask patients to place their right heel on their left shin and to slide it down and up the shin, and then to repeat the test using the left heel.

If there is an intention tremor or dysmetria (irregular error in the distance and force of limb movements), cerebellar pathologies can be investigated by looking for dysdiadochokinesis. Ask patients to slap one palm

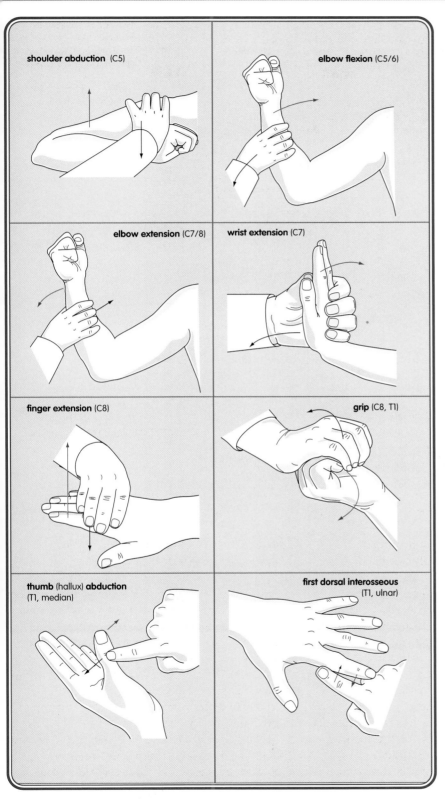

Fig. 16.13 The major muscle groups tested in an assessment of power in the upper limb. Patients should be at a slight mechanical advantage so that, if they have normal power of that muscle group, they can just overcome the resistance offered by the examiner.

shoulder abduction (C5)

elbow flexion (C5/6)

elbow extension (C7/8)

wrist extension (C7)

finger extension (C8)

grip (C8, T1)

thumb (hallux) abduction (T1, median)

first dorsal interosseous (T1, ulnar)

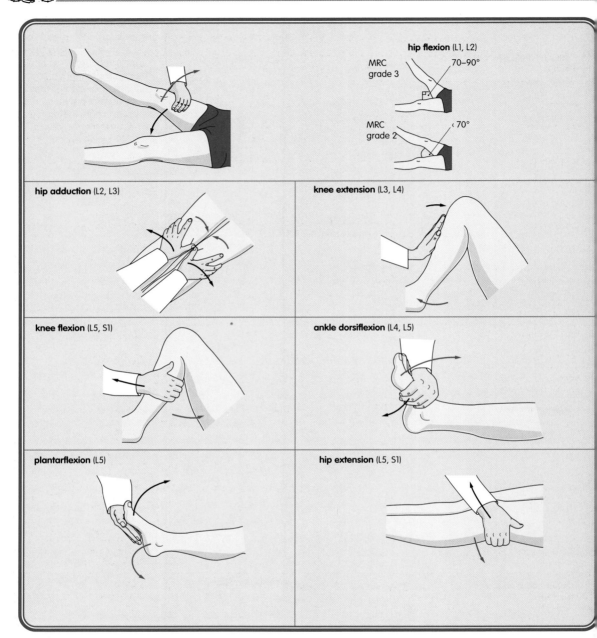

Fig. 16.14 Testing muscle groups of the lower limb.

Nerve root, peripheral nerve, and muscle responsible for each movement			
Movement	**Myotome**	**Peripheral nerve**	**Main muscle groups**
shoulder abduction	C5,6	axillary	deltoid
shoulder adduction	C5,6,7,8	lateral pectoral thoracodorsal	pectoralis major latissimus dorsi
elbow flexion	C5,6	musculocutaneous	biceps
elbow extension	C6,7,8	radial	triceps
wrist extension	C7,8	radial	long extensors
wrist flexion	C8	ulnar and median	long flexors
pronation	C6,7	median	pronator teres pronator quadratus
supination	C6,7	musculocutaneuos radial	biceps supinator
finger abduction	T1	ulnar	dorsal interossei
finger adduction	T1	ulnar	
opposition of thumb	T1	median	opponens pollicis
extension of thumb at the interphalangeal joint	T1	radial	extensor pollicis longus
hip extension	L4,5	inferior gluteal	glutei
hip flexion	L2,3	femoral	iliopsoas
knee flexion	L5,S1	sciatic	hamstrings
knee extension	L2,3,4	femoral	quadriceps
dorsiflexion of foot	L4,5	peroneal	tibialis anterior long extensors peroneus extensor digitorum brevis
plantar flexion of foot	S1,2	tibial	gastrocnemius tibialis posterior
inversion of ankle	L4	peroneal tibial	tibialis anterior tibialis posterior
eversion of ankle	S1	peroneal	peronei long extensors extensor digitorum brevis
extension of great toe	L4,5,S1	deep peroneal	extensor hallucis longus

Fig. 16.15 Nerve root, peripheral nerve, and muscle responsible for each movement. By integrating the pattern of weakness, it should be possible to recognize a pattern corresponding to these anatomical subdivisions.

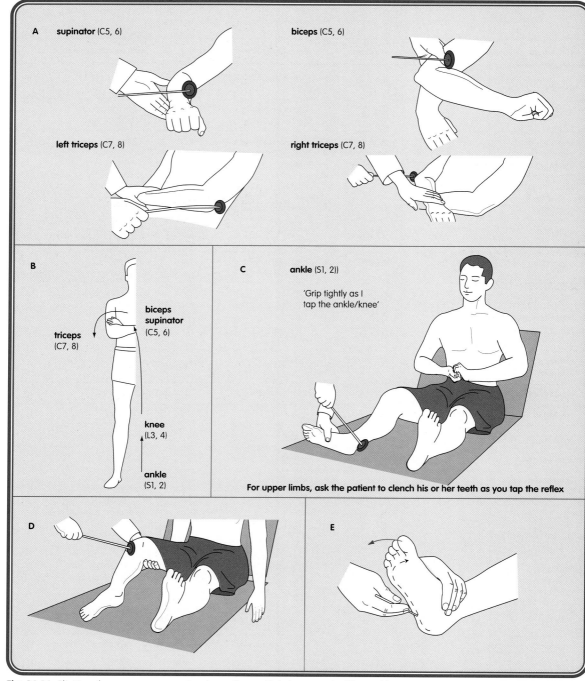

Fig. 16.16 Eliciting the more common tendon reflexes. Reinforcement of the ankle reflex is illustrated. (A) Reflexes of the upper limb. (B) Nerve roots of the tendon reflexes. (C) The ankle tendon reflex. If a reflex is difficult to elicit, reinforcement should be attempted before saying that the reflex is absent. (D) The knee reflex. (E) The plantar response.

Nerve roots supplying the major reflexes	
Reflex	**Nerve root**
biceps	C5*, C6
brachioradialis	C6*, C7
triceps	C6, C7*, C8
knee	L2, 3*, 4*
ankle	S1, S2
anal	S2, 3, 4

Fig. 16.17 Nerve roots supplying the major reflexes.
* indicates the major nerve root supplying each reflex.

rapidly with the other hand, alternating between the palm and back of the hand.

Assessment of gait

At a basic level, gait should be assessed as the patient walks into the examination room. Certain gaits are characteristic of certain pathologies. For example:

- Spastic gait—the extensor muscles are stiff and the foot is plantarflexed so patients have a stiff gait and avoid catching their toes on the ground by circumducting the leg at the hips.
- Ataxia—the gait is wide-based and there is also marked clumsiness when patients are asked to walk in

a straight line placing their heel immediately in front of the toe of the opposite foot (e.g. in cerebellar ataxia).
- High-stepping gait—in patients with footdrop, the foot is lifted high off the ground and then slapped back down.
- Parkinsonism—the gait is slow and shuffling and there is no associated arm swinging; patients often find it difficult to stop and turn around.
- Waddling gait—for example due to proximal myopathy.

No neurological assessment is complete without an assessment of the patient's gait.

Sensory system

Patients are usually aware of numbness, paraesthesiae, or altered sensation indicating a sensory pathology, but examination of the sensory system forms part of a routine assessment. Attempt to identify the modality of sensory loss and its distribution (e.g. correlating with a dermatome,

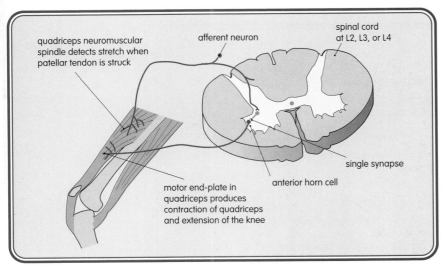

Fig. 16.18 Neurological pathway for the knee jerk.

quadriceps neuromuscular spindle detects stretch when patellar tendon is struck

afferent neuron

spinal cord at L2, L3, or L4

single synapse

anterior horn cell

motor end-plate in quadriceps produces contraction of quadriceps and extension of the knee

147

peripheral nerve). A knowledge of the dermatomes is essential (Fig. 16.19).

Light touch

Dab (do not stroke) the skin lightly with a small wisp of cotton wool. If there is decreased sensation, this should be mapped out. Start from the area of decreased sensation and move outwards as this is more sensitive.

Pin prick

Use a disposable pin or needle gently and check that the patient can identify the stimulus as sharp. Temperature sensation is also conveyed in the spinothalamic tracts, so is not usually routinely assessed.

Vibration

Place the base of a vibrating 128 Hz tuning fork on the distal phalanx of the great toe. Patients should be aware of a buzzing sensation. Ask patients to close their eyes and to indicate when they think that the tuning fork has stopped vibrating. Vibration sense is more likely to be impaired peripherally. If absent, move proximally (i.e. from lateral malleolus to upper tibia and then iliac crest).

Loss of vibration sense is one of the earlier physical signs indicative of peripheral neuropathy in diabetes mellitus.

Joint position sense

Start distally. Move the great toe passively either extending or flexing, and observe whether the patient can identify the direction of movement. Be careful not to contact the second toe with your hand as this may give additional sensation to the patient. If there is impairment, test the ankle and knee.

Romberg's test

Romberg's test may be positive if there is impaired position sense. Patients are asked to stand upright with their eyes closed. Marked swaying when patients close their eyes is Rombergism (Fig. 16.20).

Higher functions

There are many sophisticated tests of mental function. A crude screening test is the mini-mental test (Fig. 16.21). This may reveal the presence of dementia and is an essential part of any examination of an elderly person. Furthermore, a change in mental functioning may be identified over a period of time.

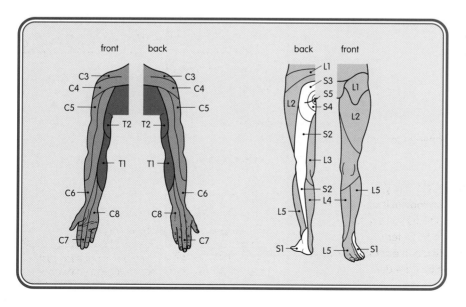

Fig. 16.19 Distribution of the dermatomes on the surface of the body.

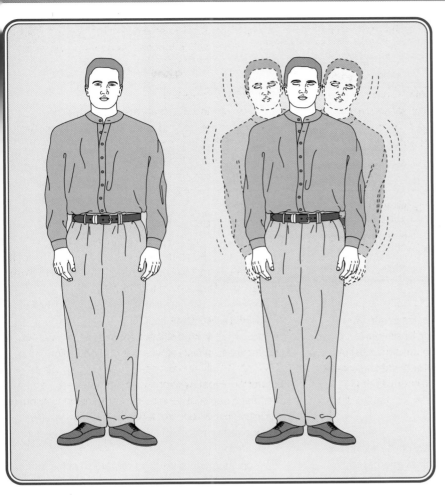

Fig. 16.20 Romberg's test. A positive test indicates impaired position sense. Patients can maintain a good posture when their eyes are open, but sway when asked to close their eyes.

Other tests should include:
- State of consciousness.
- Emotional state.
- Speech (e.g. to reveal receptive or expressive dysphasia).

If a cortical lesion is suspected, attempt to localize it (Fig. 16.22).

Patterns of neurological damage

It is helpful when assessing neurological lesions to be aware of common patterns of deficits so that the anatomical site of the lesion can be determined (e.g. myopathy, peripheral neuropathy, nerve root, cortical). Some of the more important lesions are described below.

Mini-mental test
1. time of day (to nearest hour)
2. year
3. age
4. birthday
5. place
6. recognize two people
7. dates of Second World War
8. name of the monarch
9. count backwards from 20 to 1 with no mistakes
10. recall an address given five minutes earlier

Fig. 16.21 The mini-mental test. Score one point for each correct answer. Scores of less than seven indicate well-established dementia.

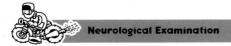
Fig. 16.22 Typical features of localized cortical lesions.

Lobe affected	Features
frontal lobe	predominant mood and behavioural changes; disinhibition; motor cortex may be involved; pout reflex
temporal lobe	dominant: sensory dysphasia, alexia (agraphia); non-dominant: may cause visuospatial deficits
parietal lobe (dominant)	aphasia; dysgraphia; dyslexia; right–left disorientation
parietal lobe (non-dominant)	neglect of contralateral sensation; altered body image; dressing apraxia; constructional apraxia

Typical features of localized cortical lesions

Myopathy

Weakness and wasting of muscles occurs in a distribution that is characteristic of the particular type of myopathy (e.g. facioscapulohumeral muscular dystrophy, Duchenne's muscular dystrophy). Reflexes are preserved until the disease is advanced.

Peripheral nerves

Radial nerve

Damage to the radial nerve may cause wrist drop. Test sensation over the first dorsal interosseous muscle (see Fig. 20.5). Test extension of the interphalangeal joint of the thumb (e.g. compression neuropathy after sleeping with arm over a chair). Radial nerve damage is most commonly a compression neuropathy (e.g heavy drinkers who sleep with their arm draped over a chair).

Median nerve

Damage to the median nerve (e.g. carpal tunnel syndrome) characteristically produces:
- Sensory loss over the palmar aspect of the lateral three and a half fingers (see Fig. 20.5).
- Wasting of the thenar eminence.
- Weakness of opposition, flexion, and abduction of the thumb.

Ulnar nerve

Ulnar nerve lesions (e.g. due to trauma at the elbow) result in:

- Sensory loss over the little finger and medial half of the ring finger (see Fig. 20.5).
- Wasting of the hypothenar eminence.
- Weakness of finger abduction and adduction.

Lateral popliteal nerve

The lateral popliteal nerve is sometimes damaged during a fracture to the head of the fibula. This may result in:
- Impaired sensation of the lateral calf.
- Footdrop.
- Weakness of dorsiflexion and eversion of the foot.

Peripheral neuropathy

Generalized neuropathy is usually in a 'stocking and glove' distribution. Tendon reflexes are lost early in the course of disease.

Cerebellum

The main features of cerebellar pathology are:
- Gait ataxia (wide-based).
- Intention tremor.
- Dysdiadochokinesis.
- Nystagmus.
- Hypotonia.
- Dysmetria.
- Dysarthria ('staccato speech').

Extrapyramidal system

There is a wide range of extrapyramidal syndromes. They tend to be characterized by:

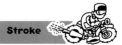

- Decreased movement (e.g. bradykinesia in Parkinson's disease).
- Involuntary movements (e.g. tardive dyskinesia with drug therapy).
- Rigidity.

Summary of neurological examination

In summary, when carrying out a neurological examination:

- It is of paramount importance to be systematic. Most of the signs represent a qualitative change from normality. This can be recognized only with practice.
- Identifying a lesion is the easy part. A given lesion may be due to multiple pathologies at various locations in the nervous system. The next stage is to prepare a list of all the elicited signs and consider whether a single pathological lesion could account for them. If so, identify its anatomical site.
- Remember that lesions produce characteristic patterns of physical signs. For example, if a weakness is identified, consider whether the pattern fits into an UMN or LMN pattern. If it is LMN, look for features that identify the site of the lesion (i.e. at the muscle itself, the neuromuscular junction, a peripheral nerve, a nerve root, or anterior horn cells). If the lesion is UMN in pattern, there are usually other localizing signs that allow identification of the anatomical point of pathology.
- Once the anatomical location of the lesion has been identified, prepare a differential diagnosis of possible pathologies that could produce a lesion at that site. Consider collateral information from the history or systemic examination to narrow down the differential diagnosis.

STROKE

Usually a diagnosis of stroke is apparent from the history, but the examination is crucial to confirm the presence of a focal neurological deficit, to document baseline function objectively, and to consider aetiological factors.

Assess level of consciousness

See section on the unconscious patient (p. 155).

Define the neurological deficit

A full neurological assessment is essential to ascertain the degree of damage. It is often possible to identify the vascular territory affected (see p. 61 and Fig. 7.8). Strokes typically result in a focal weakness, but occasionally the lesion produces a more subtle lesion such as impaired cognition. The anatomical site of damage may offer prognostic information.

Consider aetiology

The systemic examination may offer clues to the underlying cause.

Pulse

Arrhythmias, especially atrial fibrillation, predispose to emboli. Consider the possibility of a recent myocardial infarction, which may have caused a watershed infarct or have been complicated by transient arrhythmias.

Blood pressure

Hypertension is one of the major risk factors for stroke. In the acute setting, it should be interpreted with caution and treated even more cautiously, as an abrupt drop in blood pressure may cause further ischaemia as autoregulation will be impaired.

Eyes

Argyll Robertson pupils may suggest syphilis (now a rare cause of stroke in the UK) or diabetes mellitus.

Fundoscopy

Look for evidence of hypertensive and diabetic retinopathy.

Face

The facial appearance may suggest an underlying pathology, for example plethora (polycythaemia), mitral facies.

Neck

Listen carefully for a carotid bruit as a source of embolus. Have a low threshold for considering a Doppler scan of the carotid vessels as a patient with over 70% stenosis of the internal carotid artery may benefit from subsequent endarterectomy. Although detection of carotid bruits is not particularly sensitive, it is highly specific for the probability of significant stenosis.

Heart

Listen for any murmurs. Mitral stenosis (especially in association with atrial fibrillation) is a potent risk factor for left atrial thrombus and subsequent embolus. Consider the possibility of endocarditis (especially if there is a murmur). If there is fixed splitting of the second heart sound in association with a flow murmur (suggestive of an atrial communication), look for sources of paradoxical embolus from the venous circulation.

EPILEPTIC FIT

The diagnosis of epilepsy usually relies upon an objective eyewitness account. The doctor rarely sees a fit in an individual patient.

Acute seizure

The priority is to ensure that patients do not harm themselves, and then to assess and, if necessary, provide specific therapy for the fit. One should:

- Protect the airway.
- Ensure that the patient will not harm him or herself.
- Observe the nature of the seizure activity (e.g. tonic–clonic, focal, absence attack).
- Check pulse rate and, if possible, blood pressure.
- Check blood sugar, obtain blood for electrolytes (toxins).
- If fit is prolonged, treat as for status epilepticus.

Postictal

Usually the patient is seen in the postictal period, having been brought to hospital after collapsing. The history is central to the diagnosis (see 'Presenting complaints', p. 58), and very often the examination is unremarkable. The examination may be useful when considering the differential diagnosis or for assessing the aetiology and functional consequences of the fit (Fig. 16.23).

Perform detailed neurological assessment

In particular, focus on:

- Level of consciousness. Check the Glasgow coma score (see Fig. 16.24) until a normal level of consciousness is achieved, as seizure may be the presentation of head injury or intracranial bleed.
- Paralysis. A postictal focal weakness (Todd's paralysis) may be present for 24 hours following a fit, but consider the presence of an acute CVA or intracranial space-occupying lesion if neurological signs are present.
- Eyes. Check pupillary responses and fundoscopy to exclude papilloedema.

Perform systemic examination to identify precipitating cause

It is particularly important to perform a detailed systemic examination to try to identify an underlying cause for the epileptic fit so that specific therapy may be offered. Consider:

Assessment of a patient during a 'fit' to reveal conditions other than typical epilepsy	
Cause of collapse	**Discriminatory features**
syncope	usually apparent from prodromal history check pulse rate (e.g. tachyarrhythmia, Stokes–Adams attack) check postural blood pressure pallor during episode
narcolepsy	no convulsions patient rousable
hysteria	often many atypical features usually occur only where there is an audience no urinary incontinence/tongue biting

Fig. 16.23 Assessment of a patient during a 'fit' may reveal the presence of a condition other than typical epilepsy.

- Alcohol withdrawal—signs of chronic liver disease, smell of alcohol on breath, unkempt condition, common.
- Trauma.
- Pyrexia—infants.
- Encephalitis—fever, level of consciousness, focal neurological signs, herpetic ulcer.
- Malignancy—look for signs of primary bronchial, breast, colonic, or kidney tumour.
- Degenerative brain disease (e.g. dementia).

UNCONSCIOUS PATIENT

Assessment of the unconscious patient provides a great challenge for the diagnostic and management skills of the physician. The first priority is to ensure that the patient is stable before performing a detailed assessment. As always, assess the basic parameters first:
- Airway. Check that it is patent, and the patient is able to protect it.
- Breathing and pulse. Check the carotid pulse. If absent, initiate cardiopulmonary resuscitation.
- Circulation and blood pressure. If hypotensive, look for and treat causes of shock (especially trauma).

Assess level of consciousness

The Glasgow coma score is widely used to provide a simple reproducible objective assessment of conscious level. This is based on the best responses obtained (Fig. 16.24).

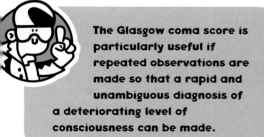

The Glasgow coma score is particularly useful if repeated observations are made so that a rapid and unambiguous diagnosis of a deteriorating level of consciousness can be made.

Perform full neurological examination

Look for any localizing signs. Pay particular attention to:
- Pupil size and response to light (Fig. 16.25) (including symmetry)—some drugs (e.g. opiates) constrict pupils; other drugs (e.g. phenothiazines, amphetamines) dilate pupils; 'coning' results in a single fixed dilated pupil; pontine lesion results in pin-point pupils; brain death results in fixed dilated pupils.
- Fundi (especially for papilloedema).
- Gag and corneal reflexes.
- Doll's eye reflexes.
- Motor responses.
- Tendon reflexes.
- Abnormal tone.

Perform detailed systemic examination

Coma may be due to metabolic, infective, cardiovascular wide ranging pathology (e.g metabolic, infective cardiovascular lesions). In particular, note:
- Evidence of trauma or head injury (look for otorrhoea or cerebrospinal fluid leaking from the nose).
- Temperature (e.g. hyperthermia may be due to hypothyroidism, fever may be due to infection).
- Evidence of needle marks (indicating diabetes mellitus or drug addiction).
- Jaundice or other features of chronic liver disease.
- Breath (e.g. revealing hepatic foetor, alcohol, diabetic ketoacidosis).

Glasgow coma score	
eyes (E)	
open spontaneously (with blinking)	4
open to command or speech	3
open in response to pain (applied to limbs or sternum)	2
not opening	1
motor function (M)	
obeys commands	6
localizes to pain	5
withdraws from pain	4
flexor response to pain (decorticate)	3
extensor response to pain (decerebrate)	2
no response to pain	1
vocalization (V)	
appropriate speech	5
confused speech	4
inappropriate words	3
groans only	2
no speech	1

Fig. 16.24 Glasgow coma score.

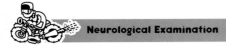
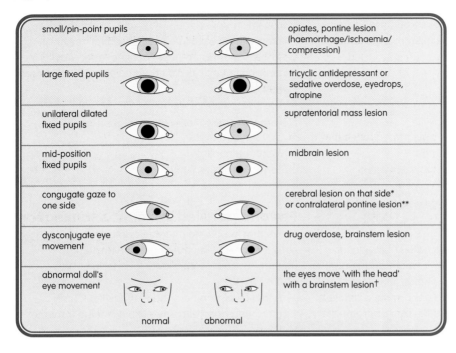

small/pin-point pupils			opiates, pontine lesion (haemorrhage/ischaemia/ compression)
large fixed pupils			tricyclic antidepressant or sedative overdose, eyedrops, atropine
unilateral dilated fixed pupils			supratentorial mass lesion
mid-position fixed pupils			midbrain lesion
congugate gaze to one side			cerebral lesion on that side* or contralateral pontine lesion**
dysconjugate eye movement			drug overdose, brainstem lesion
abnormal doll's eye movement	normal	abnormal	the eyes move 'with the head' with a brainstem lesion†

Fig. 16.25 Examination of the pupils in an unconscious patient. Note the size and reaction to light. In addition, note the position of gaze fixation. (*Looking towards the lesion; **looking away from the lesion; †normally if the head is held and turned quickly from side to side the eyes swivel in the opposite direction to the head.)

- Respiratory pattern (e.g. Cheyne–Stokes respiration, Kussmaul's respiration of diabetic ketoacidosis or uraemia).
- Cyanosis (e.g. due to hypoxia).

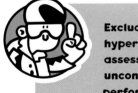

Exclude hypoglycaemia or hyperglycaemia early in the assessment of an unconscious patient by performing a BM stick analysis.

MULTIPLE SCLEROSIS

Multiple sclerosis causes neurological lesions that are disseminated in time and place. It can be diagnosed with reasonable confidence from the history of relapses and remissions and thorough examination if it follows a typical course. Areas of demyelination may occur anywhere in the central nervous system, but certain patterns are more common.

Sites of involvement
The more common sites of involvement are:
- Optic nerve (optic neuritis).

- Brainstem.
- Cerebellum.
- Cervical cord.
- Periventricular region.

Eyes
Certain patterns of disease should be distinguished, for example:
- Retrobulbar neuritis—relative afferent pupillary defect (inappropriate dilatation of one pupil when shining a light directly into one eye and then the other), central scotoma.
- Optic neuritis—also note swelling of the optic disc acutely, and temporal pallor following recovery.
- Optic atrophy—this is a common finding in long-standing multiple sclerosis, but should be distinguished from other pathologies (Fig. 16.26).
- Nystagmus—often jerking or ataxic; pronounced in late disease.
- Internuclear ophthalmoplegia—diplopia on lateral gaze due to failure of adducting eye to cross midline and demyelination of medial longitudinal bundle.

Brainstem
Multiple brainstem or cerebellar signs may be present, especially nystagmus, diplopia, intention tremor, scanning speech.

Spinal cord

Spastic paraparesis is common in late disease. Other signs can include bladder dysfunction, decreased limb sensation, and loss of posture sensibility, which is often marked.

Mental

Both euphoria and depression or irritability are common.

Always attempt to make a functional assessment of how multiple sclerosis might affect daily activities.

Differential diagnosis of optic atrophy	
Site of lesion	**Causes**
retina	central retinal occlusion toxic (e.g. quinine, methylated spirits)
optic nerve	optic and retrobulbar neuritis, (e.g. multiple sclerosis) chronic glaucoma any cause of papilloedema toxin (e.g. alcohol, tobacco, ethambutol) tumour (e.g. meningioma, optic glioma)
optic chiasm	pituitary tumours craniopharyngioma meningioma,

Fig. 16.26 Differential diagnosis of optic atrophy.

Inspection

Note weight as diabetic control may improve with weight reduction.

Macrovascular complications

Ischaemic heart disease and cerebrovascular disease

Diabetics have a much increased risk of stroke and ischaemic heart disease. It is important to modify any reversible risk factors. Assess these other risk factors, especially:

- Obesity—obesity is not only a risk factor for macrovascular disease, but predisposes to poor glycaemic control.
- Blood pressure control.
- Smoking—nicotine staining of fingers and hair.
- Xanthoma, arcus senilis.

Peripheral vascular disease

Examine the peripheral pulses (femoral, popliteal, dorsalis pedis and posterior tibial arteries). Consider measuring the ratio of ankle:brachial artery pressure. Listen for bruits, especially over the abdomen and carotid and femoral arteries, which indicate turbulent flow and are suggestive of stenosis.

Look for evidence of ulcers, including between the toes. Ulcers may be painless and , although large, patients may be unaware of them.

Microvascular complications

Eyes

Examination of the eyes is important in diabetic patients as they are at risk of many diseases. Diabetic patients should have a detailed fundoscopic assessment with dilated pupils at least once a year. Note the following:

- Cataracts—these are more common in diabetics.
- Evidence of background retinopathy ('dot and blot' haemorrhages, exudates).
- Proliferative retinopathy (neovascularization, vitreous haemorrhage).
- Macular oedema.

Assess eye movements (especially in long-standing diabetes mellitus) for a third nerve palsy due to mononeuritis multiplex.

Check visual acuity, which is often reduced due to maculopathy.

Peripheral neuropathy

Test for evidence of a 'stocking and glove' sensory loss. Loss of vibration and joint position sense are often the first modalities to be affected, especially in the legs. A defined peripheral nerve (e.g. median nerve) lesion (mononeuritis multiplex) may also be present.

Diabetic nephropathy

Nephropathy is particularly common in the presence of retinopathy and neuropathy. It is also a marker for an increased risk of ischaemic heart disease. Look for proteinuria and microbinuria at every annual assessment.

Urinalysis is an essential component of examination of the diabetic patient!

Feet

The feet of diabetic patients should be examined at every examination. Look at general foot care such as the presence of ulcers and the state of the nails. Test the temperature, pulses, and shape of the foot to determine vascular and neuropathic causes of any ulceration. The presence of abnormally sited callosities on the sole may indicate uneven weight distribution.

Assess diabetic control

Different patients use different methods for recording glucose control.

Urinalysis

Look for glycosuria, but be aware of the different renal thresholds for glycosuria. If a patient consistently has negative glycosuria, it may be worth checking a level of glycosylated haemoglobin (HbA$_{IC}$).

Blood glucose
Look at the patient's own record of blood glucose stick assessments. This is most informative in type I diabetes mellitus. You may wish to ask patients to perform an estimate in front of you so that you can assess their technique.

Evidence of skin infections (e.g. boils, abscesses, candidiasis) may suggest chronically poor control.

Assessing injection sites
Look for complications such as scarring, abscesses, and lipodystrophy, which result from not rotating injection sites frequently enough.

Diabetic coma
A young patient presenting with diabetes may present with diabetic ketoacidosis. Any treated patient may have hypoglycaemia complicating therapy.

If there is any doubt about the cause of a coma in a diabetic patient and the glucose level is not known, treat with intravenous glucose first.

Diabetic ketoacidosis
This typically occurs in a child or young adult. In particular:
- Note the respiratory pattern—Kussmaul's respiration suggests acidosis ('air hunger').
- Note the mental state—may be alert, but usually confused or stuporose.
- Smell the breath—ketones may be detectable.
- Consider fluid status—the patient is invariably dehydrated with dry skin and mucous membranes, decreased (or undetectable) jugular venous pressure (JVP), and hypotension.
- Consider the underlying cause.
- Fever is often absent before therapy, even in the presence of infection, but sources of infection should be carefully sought.

Hyperosmolar non-ketotic coma
Hyperosmolar non-ketotic coma usually presents in a fashion similar to that in diabetic ketoacidosis, but in elderly and middle-aged subjects. Many of the clinical signs are the same, as are the basic management strategies, as follows:
- Rehydrate.
- Optimize acid–base balance.
- Replace insulin deficiency.
- Look for and treat the underlying cause.
- Provide general supportive care.

The management of diabetic ketoacidosis and hyperosmolar non-ketotic coma differ only in the fine tuning.

HYPERTHYROIDISM

Like hypothyroidism (see below), many systems may show signs of hyperthyroidism, and although marked hyperthyroidism due to Graves' disease is unmistakable, the signs are often non-specific, and hyperthyroidism occurs in the differential diagnosis of many symptoms and signs.

Inspection
General inspection often provides clues that are easily overlooked (Fig. 17.1). In particular, note:
- General demeanour—patients are typically agitated, restless, irritable, and have poor concentration.
- Facies.
- Goitre—associated with Graves' disease, toxic multinodular goitre.

Cardiovascular system
Cardiovascular abnormalities are common in thyroid disease and may provide a sensitive measure of assessing thyroid status in a treated patient. Look for the presence of:
- Tachycardia—very common.
- Atrial fibrillation—although this is a common arrhythmia, its presence should always raise a suspicion of hyperthyroidism—this is important as hyperthyroidism is an easily treatable cause of this arrhythmia.

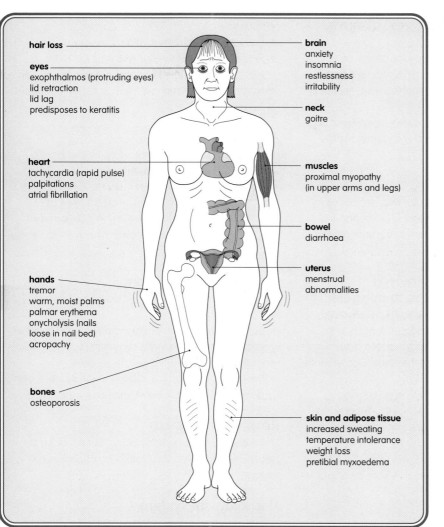

Fig. 17.1 Symptoms and signs of hyperthyroidism.

hair loss

eyes
exophthalmos (protruding eyes)
lid retraction
lid lag
predisposes to keratitis

heart
tachycardia (rapid pulse)
palpitations
atrial fibrillation

hands
tremor
warm, moist palms
palmar erythema
onycholysis (nails
loose in nail bed)
acropachy

bones
osteoporosis

brain
anxiety
insomnia
restlessness
irritability

neck
goitre

muscles
proximal myopathy
(in upper arms and legs)

bowel
diarrhoea

uterus
menstrual
abnormalities

skin and adipose tissue
increased sweating
temperature intolerance
weight loss
pretibial myxoedema

The presence of atrial fibrillation in any patient should provoke a search for the underlying cause. The most common causes are:
- **Ischaemic heart disease.**
- **Hyperthyroidism.**
- **Mitral valve disease (especially mitral stenosis).**

- Warm vasodilated peripheries with a bounding arterial pulse.
- Hypertension— occasionally a feature.

Neurological system

A brief examination often reveals discriminatory signs, for example:
- Fine resting tremor.
- Agitated, restless, hyperactive, shaky, irritable mental state. The patient may have a frank psychosis.
- Proximal myopathy, which may be profound.

Features to suggest Graves' disease
Eye signs
Graves' disease is particularly associated with eye signs, and this can be used to differentiate it from other causes of hyperthyroidism. Note the presence of:

- Lid lag—upper eyelid does not keep pace with the eyeball as it follows a finger moving downwards from above.
- Exophthalmos.
- Chemosis.
- Ophthalmoplegia —extraocular muscles become swollen and develop secondary fibrotic changes.
- Proptosis—most common cause of unilateral and bilateral proptosis.

Pretibial myxoedema, thyroid acropachy, and features to suggest general autoimmune predisposition
Deposition of mucopolysaccharides in the subcutaneous tissues of the legs produces a non-tender infiltration on the front of the shins. Occasionally, it can present acutely.

Thyroid acropachy is a syndrome resembling clubbing with new bone formation in the fingers. It is classically associated with exophthalmos and pretibial myxoedema.

Thyroid disease is associated with other autoimmune processes. In particular, look for alopecia and vitiligo.

HYPOTHYROIDISM

Hypothyroidism often develops insidiously and non-specifically, especially in the elderly. A keen level of awareness is important, and the diagnosis is often made by an observant doctor who has never seen the patient previously.

Inspection
It is easy to overlook hypothyroidism, so always consider the diagnosis, especially for patients presenting with chronic fatigue, dementia, slow thought, or non-specific difficulty in coping with previously simple tasks (Fig. 17.2). Note the:

- Facies.
- Body shape—obesity, which is usually mild.
- Presence of a goitre—for example if due to Hashimoto's thyroiditis, iodine deficiency.
- Non-pitting oedema.

It is very easy to overlook a diagnosis of hypothyroidism. Always maintain a high index of suspicion, especially if the patient is seen on a regular basis.

Cardiovascular system
Discriminatory features may include:
- Cold peripheries.
- Bradycardia—a useful sign, especially if it is out of context with the patient's condition.
- Hypothermia.
- Pericardial effusion (i.e. difficult to locate apex beat, quiet heart sounds), heart failure.

Respiratory system
There are rarely any specific signs, but check for a pleural effusion—a transudate is an uncommon feature.

Neurological system
It is common to find neurological signs, for example:
- Slow-relaxing deep tendon reflexes.
- Proximal myopathy.
- Carpal tunnel syndrome.
- Deep, hoarse voice.
- Mental slowing, which may present with dementia, stupor, or even coma.

Slow-relaxing reflexes are a particularly useful sign for confirming a clinical suspicion of hypothyroidism.

Fig. 17.2 Symptoms and signs of hypothyroidism.

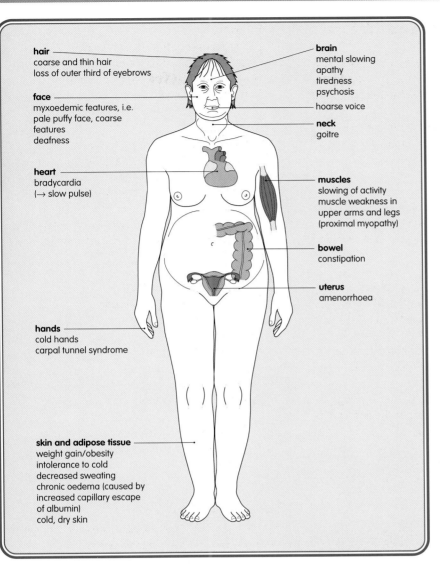

hair
coarse and thin hair
loss of outer third of eyebrows

face
myxoedemic features, i.e.
pale puffy face, coarse
features
deafness

heart
bradycardia
(→ slow pulse)

hands
cold hands
carpal tunnel syndrome

skin and adipose tissue
weight gain/obesity
intolerance to cold
decreased sweating
chronic oedema (caused by
increased capillary escape
of albumin)
cold, dry skin

brain
mental slowing
apathy
tiredness
psychosis

hoarse voice

neck
goitre

muscles
slowing of activity
muscle weakness in
upper arms and legs
(proximal myopathy)

bowel
constipation

uterus
amenorrhoea

18. Reticulo-endothelial Examination

Examination of lymph node groups is important in many disease states. Learn the anatomical drainage pattern of the major organs as regional lymphadenopathy may be the first manifestation of local disease.

Normally, lymph nodes are not palpable, except in some thin people. If a single lymph node is found to be enlarged, it is important to adopt a systematic approach.

EXAMINATION ROUTINE

Examine all lymph node groups

Examine all the lymph node groups systematically to define the anatomical distribution of the enlarged lymph nodes (Fig. 18.1). It is important to examine the liver and spleen as well, as these are also reticuloendothelial organs and may be enlarged in the presence of generalized lymphadenopathy.

Define the characteristics of the enlarged lymph node(s)

Define the texture, size, mobility, and fixation to superficial and other tissues of the enlarged lymph node(s) (as with the examination of any lump). Certain characteristics are suggestive of different disease processes. For example:

- Rubbery texture is suggestive of lymphoma.
- Hard, matted, fixed lymph nodes suggest malignancy.
- Tender lymph nodes suggest infection or other inflammatory state.

Explore the region drained by the enlarged lymph node group

If a single lymph node group is enlarged, try to identify the cause. The broad causes of lymphadenopathy are:

- Infection.
- Metastatic tumour.
- Lymphoproliferative disorder.
- Sarcoidosis.

In cases of cellulitis or other bacterial infection, it is sometimes possible to see lymphangitis. It is visible as thin red streaks following the line of the lymphatics in the skin.

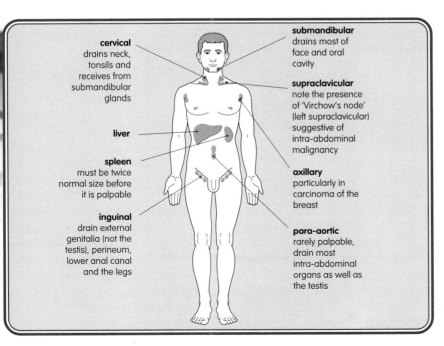

cervical
drains neck, tonsils and receives from submandibular glands

liver

spleen
must be twice normal size before it is palpable

inguinal
drain external genitalia (not the testis), perineum, lower anal canal and the legs

submandibular
drains most of face and oral cavity

supraclavicular
note the presence of 'Virchow's node' (left supraclavicular) suggestive of intra-abdominal malignancy

axillary
particularly in carcinoma of the breast

para-aortic
rarely palpable, drain most intra-abdominal organs as well as the testis

Fig. 18.1 Position of the major lymph node groups and lymphoid organs.

Perform a systemic examination

Consider the pathological cause by performing a systemic examination, concentrating on inflammatory or malignant conditions draining into that lymph node group.

Consider the more common causes of localized and systemic lymphadenopathy (Fig. 18.2).

Usually, the cause of lymphadenopathy is apparent from a detailed history and systemic examination, but if further investigation is needed, the most useful tests include:

- Full blood count and film—for infection, leukaemia.
- Erythrocyte sedimentation rate (ESR) and C-reactive protein (CRP)—for malignancy, systemic inflammatory disease, systemic lupus erythematosus (SLE)—these are markers of an acute inflammatory response, and a differential rise in ESR or CRP is occasionally discriminatory.
- Biochemical profile, especially liver function.
- Chest radiography—for example for sarcoid, malignancy, chest infection.
- Viral screens, autoantibody profiles, blood culture.
- Lymph node biopsy—often provides diagnostic information if sinister pathology is suspected.

If a single lymph node is enlarged, explore the region drained by that lymph node in detail.

Regional lymphadenopathy is common, but usually transient. Persistent lymphadenopathy always warrants investigation.

		Differential diagnosis of localized and generalized lymphadenopathy	
	Lymphadenopathy	**Features and examples**	
localized	infection (bacterial, viral, fungal)	pharyngitis, dental (cervical); lymphogranuloma venereum (inguinal)	
	lymphoma (Hodgkin's; non-Hodgkin's)	can present anywhere, but cervical group is the most common	
	malignancy	Virchow's node (left supraclavicular lymphadenopathy due to intra-abdominal or thoracic disease); breast cancer (axillary or supraclavicular)	
generalized	infection	infectious mononucleosis; syphilis; tuberculosis; toxoplasmosis; HIV	
	malignancy	lymphoma; leukaemia (especially CLL); carcinoma (unusual)	
	autoimmune disease	SLE, rheumatoid arthritis, sarcoidosis, other connective tissue diseases	
	drugs		
	hyperthyroidism		

Fig. 18.2 Differential diagnosis of localized and generalized lymphadenopathy. (CLL, chronic lymphocytic leukaemia; SLE, systemic lupus erythematosus.)

19. Breast Examination

EXAMINATION ROUTINE

Breast examination forms an integral part of a full medical clerking. However, a more detailed breast examination is always necessary if the presenting symptoms include the following:

- Breast symptoms (e.g. lump, pain, nipple discharge, change in appearance).
- Suspicion of disseminated malignancy with an undiagnosed primary (e.g. presentation with pleural effusion, hepatomegaly, bony tenderness).
- Fever of unknown cause.

As with any system, a methodical approach is needed. Anticipate what information might be obtained from each part of the examination and how each elicited sign is placed into context with the presenting illness.

Patient exposure and position

Clearly, great sensitivity is essential. Very often the patient feels uncomfortable or embarrassed, especially if the doctor is male. Remember that many patients will be terrified, not only of the examination but of the potential underlying diagnosis. It is not uncommon for women to 'ignore' a breast mass for several months or even years.

Explain clearly why the examination is being performed and the useful information that is likely to be gained. Ensure complete privacy. It is clearly unacceptable for a secretary or another doctor to burst through the door revealing a semi-clad patient to the waiting room! The room should be warm, and a blanket should always be provided so that the patient can remain covered until the examination is performed.

Explain clearly what the examination will entail before asking the patient to undress. Ask the patient to remove all clothing (including bra) from the waist upwards, and to sit on the side of the examination couch. The patient should be given the option of having a chaperone if she wishes and if one is available.

The examination follows the usual sequence of:

- Inspection.
- Palpation.
- Systemic examination.

Inspection

Remember to look at the whole patient. Make a mental note of:

- Age. Breast carcinoma is more common in older women, but can occur in any age group from the third decade onwards. Fibroadenoma is more common in premenopausal women. Abscess is much more common in women of childbearing age.
- Sex. Men also get breast disease!
- General health.

Breast substance

Ask patients to sit still facing you with their arms by their side (Fig. 19.1), and with their arms raised above their head—a mass tethered to the skin may then become apparent, and the undersurface of the breasts can be seen. Note:

- Symmetry. It is not uncommon for one breast to be slightly larger than the other, but underlying masses, infections, or nipple disease can also cause asymmetry of size, shape, or nipples.
- Any obvious mass.
- Skin discolouration. Infections and occasionally malignancy may cause a red discolouration.
- Skin puckering or peau d'orange (Fig. 19.2). Peau d'orange is caused by infiltration of the skin lymphatic system and, as the name implies, its appearance resembles the peel of an orange.

Nipples

Inspect the nipples carefully, especially noting the following:

- Symmetry.
- Retraction or deviation. If one or both nipples are retracted, ask the patient if this is a new phenomenon. This is an ominous sign. As well as carcinoma, it is associated with chronic abscess and fat necrosis.

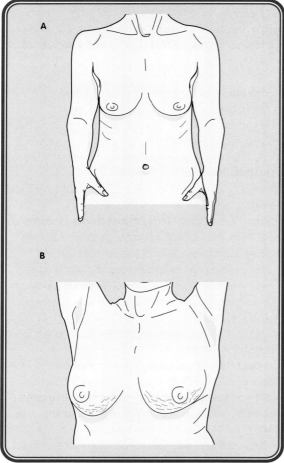

Fig. 19.1 (A) Ask the patient to sit facing you with hands on hips. (B) Then ask the patient to lift her arms in the air. Skin tethering may become apparent, and abnormalities on the undersurface of the breast will become visible.

- Discharge. If present, note whether it appears milky (galactorrhoea), bloody, or pustular.
- Skin colour. Particularly note the presence of an eczematous rash suggestive of Paget's disease of the nipple.

Palpation

The normal consistency of a breast varies considerably. It is advisable to start the examination with palpation of the normal breast. Palpate with the palmar surface of the fingers. It is helpful to divide the breast into quadrants (Fig. 19.3). Palpate each quadrant in turn, noting:

- Consistency and texture of the breast.
- Tenderness.
- Presence of any mass.

Examine the breast with symptoms. Before palpating, ask patients to point to the area of tenderness or to any lump that they may have felt. Once again, examine each quadrant in turn. If a mass is felt, it should be systematically examined as described below.

Breast mass

If any lump or mass is identified on systemic examination, the essential features should be described. This is well illustrated with a breast mass. The following characteristics should be noted.

Position

It is usual to describe a breast mass in relation to the quadrant it is located in. A breast carcinoma is more

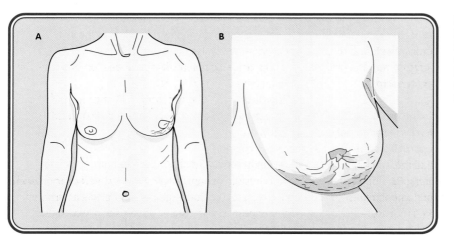

Fig. 19.2 Inspection often reveals obvious asymmetry. (A) A retracted nipple and skin tethering on the left breast. (B) Peau d'orange in association with a retracted nipple.

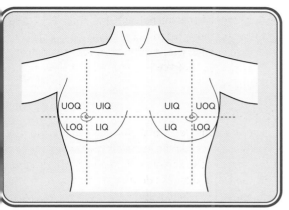

Fig. 19.3 Quadrants of the breast. Upper outer quadrant (UOQ), upper inner quadrant (UIQ), lower outer quadrant (LOQ), lower inner quadrant (LIQ).

common in the upper outer quadrant. Remember to palpate the axillary tail as this also contains breast tissue.

Size
Describe the size of the mass in two dimensions. Ideally, measure the mass objectively with a tape meaure or callipers to decrease interobserver error. This is essential when assessing the progression or regression of a lesion (e.g. judging the response of breast carcinoma to chemotherapy).

Consistency
Note the consistency of any mass. In practice, it is easiest to use terms such as:
- 'Hard'—like pressing on your forehead.
- 'Rubbery'—like pressing on the tip of your nose.
- 'Soft'—like pressing on your lips.

Relation to the skin
Note the presence of tethering or fixation to the skin. Fixation suggests an infiltrating carcinoma; tethering occurs in carcinoma, abscess, or fat necrosis.

Relation to underlying tissue
Note the mobility of any lump. A mass fixed to deeper tissue is much more likely to be a carcinoma.

Fibroadenomas are typically described as highly mobile, and may be difficult to palpate. Trapping a fibroadenoma between finger and thumb can be tricky, and has been likened to chasing a mouse, hence the term 'breast mouse'.

Tenderness
Breast carcinoma is rarely tender on presentation. A tender mass is much more likely to be an abscess, cyst, or fat necrosis.

Skin discolouration
Note any change in the appearance of the skin overlying the mass. Erythema is common in association with infections; Paget's disease of the nipple presents with an eczematous rash; a carcinoma occasionally has a red or blue hue.

Temperature
Inflammatory lesions often produce palpable warmth.

Associated lesions
It is essential to examine the rest of the breast for the presence of a second mass. It is not rare for breast carcinoma to present with bilateral disease. Fibroadenosis often presents with multiple lumps.

If breast carcinoma is suspected, a full systemic examination is essential. Look for evidence of metastatic spread. In particular, check for the presence of:
- Hepatomegaly—liver metastases result in a grim prognosis; note the presence of jaundice.
- Pleural effusion—the lung is a common site of metastatic spread.
- Bony tenderness—bony metastases are the most common site of secondary breast malignancy after axillary lymph nodes and the axial skeleton is often involved; disease may be present for several years in an otherwise relatively asymptomatic woman.
- Ascites—peritoneal deposits often present with ascites.

Lymphatic drainage
Palpation of the axillary lymph nodes forms part of the routine breast examination (see below).

An example of a recording of the presence of a breast mass in the medical notes is illustrated in Fig. 19.4.

Axillary examination
Breast examination is incomplete without examination of the axillae as these are the natural site of lymphatic drainage of breast tissue. Inspect the axillae for any obvious lumps.

167

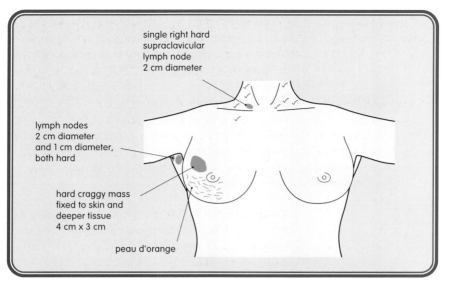

single right hard
supraclavicular
lymph node
2 cm diameter

lymph nodes
2 cm diameter
and 1 cm diameter,
both hard

hard craggy mass
fixed to skin and
deeper tissue
4 cm x 3 cm

peau d'orange

Fig. 19.4 Example of a recording of the presence of a breast mass in the medical notes. A simple diagram provides unambiguous objective information.

Axillary lymphadenopathy can be palpated only if the muscles forming the walls of the axilla are relaxed. Stand on the patient's right-hand side, support the patient's right upper arm with your right hand, and encourage the patient to allow you to take the weight of the arm (Fig. 19.5). Palpate the axilla with your left hand flat against the lateral chest wall, reaching high up into the axilla with your fingertips, sweeping around all of the walls. The left axilla is examined in a similar manner, but with the opposite hand.

If any mass is detected in the breast or axilla, the supraclavicular and cervical lymph nodes should also be examined.

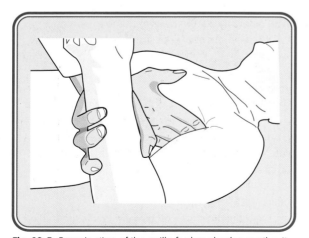

Fig. 19.5 Examination of the axilla for lymphadenopathy. It is important to support the patient's arm to relax the muscles of the axillary folds.

Finally, note the size of the patient's arms. Lymphoedema can result from tumour invasion of the lymphatics, axillary dissection, or radiotherapy.

The key to successful examination of the axilla is to ensure that the arm is totally relaxed and supported by your hand.

BREAST MASS

Presentation with a breast mass is common. Clearly, the most important diagnosis to exclude is carcinoma of the breast. The most common causes are listed below.

Carcinoma of the breast

In the presence of a breast mass, features to suggest carcinoma include:

- A hard, craggy mass.
- Fixation of the mass to skin or deeper tissues.
- Nipple deviation or retraction.
- Skin changes (peau d'orange, tethering, ulceration).
- Axillary lymphadenopathy.
- Signs of systemic disease.

Fibroadenoma

A fibroadenoma is typically a well-demarcated, highly mobile, non-tender mass in a young or middle-aged woman.

Fibroadenosis (cystic hyperplasia, fibrocystic disease)

The features of fibroadenosis are highly variable and depend upon the proportion of cystic change, fibrosis, and masses. Often there is a diffuse change in texture in the breasts and there are multiple masses, which are poorly defined. Mild tenderness is common.

Abscess

Abscesses usually present in lactating women and are easily distinguished by the presence of:

- Tenderness.
- Erythema.
- Poor definition.
- Axillary lymphadenopathy.
- Systemic features of infection (e.g fever, tachycardia).

Fat necrosis

Fat necrosis is much more common in large breasts and typically follows a history of trauma a history of trauma. The lump is usually hard and may be tethered to the skin. It may be distinguishable from a breast carcinoma by the lack of axillary lymphadenopathy or peau d'orange.

BREAST PAIN

The more common causes of breast pain are:

- Fibroadenosis.
- Premenstrual tension.
- Mastitis.
- Abscess.

The cause is usually apparent from the history and physical examination. Breast carcinoma rarely presents with pain.

GYNAECOMASTIA

Gynaecomastia results from an increase in breast tissue in males. It may be unilateral or bilateral, and is confirmed by palpation. The most common causes are:

- Puberty. Normal finding (very common).
- Old age.
- Liver failure (look for stigmata of chronic liver disease).
- Carcinoma of the lung.
- Testicular tumours.
- Adrenal tumours.
- Drugs (e.g. spironolactone, cimetidine, digoxin).
- Testicular feminization (rare).
- Pituitary tumours.

INVESTIGATIONS

The cause of many breast lesions is often apparent from a careful history and physical examination. However, in many circumstances it is important to exclude breast carcinoma. The most reliable procedure for such exclusion is to perform an excision biopsy, but it is clearly desirable for this to be avoided for benign lesions.

Mammography is performed as a screening procedure in the UK for women over 50 years of age. In the presence of a lump, mammography provides a useful adjunct to clinical examination by detecting areas of calcification, which are indicative of an underlying carcinoma. In addition, a second suspicious area may also be revealed, which should also be investigated clinically.

Ultrasound can be used to identify the composition (i.e. solid versus cystic) of a mass. Cystic lesions can be aspirated as a diagnostic or therapeutic procedure. Ultrasound is often requested to localize masses before surgery. In addition, this technique can be used to identify masses for fine needle aspiration (FNA). FNA may provide adequate cytological information to increase or decrease the clinical index of suspicion of malignancy, and so determine the urgency of treatment.

20. Locomotor Examination

EXAMINATION ROUTINE

Locomotor assessment is fundamental to even the shortest medical clerking as information on the patient's functional ability is assessed and integrated with other physical signs. Clearly, if a patient describes decreased mobility, weakness, or joint pain, a more detailed general assessment is necessary. Equally, if a focal abnormality is detected, this should be fully examined.

This chapter is not intended to provide a detailed description of examination of every joint and muscle group, but illustrates a methodical and functional approach to examining the system.

Patient exposure and position

When examining muscle groups or mobility it is important to ensure that patients are properly exposed. They should be provided with a blanket and asked to strip to their underwear in a warm, well-lit room. The initial formal assessment is usually performed on the examination couch.

Inspection

General inspection

Remember that the examination should begin as soon as the patient walks into the examination room! It is often possible to form an impression of functional ability by observing how easily the patient gets out of the chair, walks to the examination room, and climbs onto the examination couch. Note the following.

Age and sex

Different disease processes are more likely to occur at different ages, for example:
- Osteoarthritis and polymyalgia rheumatica are more common in the elderly.
- Osteoporosis is primarily a disease of postmenopausal women.
- Ankylosing spondylitis usually presents in young men.
- Many inflammatory arthritides present in young women.

Racial origin

Many forms of arthritis or diseases presenting with impaired mobility have a strong genetic predisposition and are more common in certain racial groups. Others have a predominantly environmental cause that varies geographically, for example:
- Systemic lupus erythematosus (SLE) is most common in Afro-Caribbean women.
- Tuberculous discitis is most common in patients from the Indian subcontinent.
- Paget's disease is most common in Caucasians.
- Multiple sclerosis is most common in patients from temperate climates.

General health and appearance

Note whether the patient appears well or is cachexic: obesity predisposes to osteoarthritis of the back and lower limb; cachexia may indicate chronic systemic disease or carcinoma. Note whether the patient appears to be in pain at rest or on walking. An obvious focal weakness may be apparent. These non-verbal clues may contrast with the information obtained from the history or when the patient knows that a formal examination is being performed.

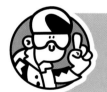

The most important part of the locomotor examination is inspection.

Facial appearance

Note the appearance of facial asymmetry or obvious weakness. In addition, note the general appearance (e.g. myopathic facies of muscular dystrophy with unlined expressionless facies and wasting of the facial muscles).

How easily does the patient get out of a chair?

Proximal muscle weakness (e.g. due to polymyalgia rheumatica, steroid myopathy, hyperthyroidism) will have a profound effect on getting up from a seated position.

Does the patient require any aids for walking?

Observe whether the patient walks unaided into the examination room or walks with the aid of a walking stick or zimmer frame, or holding on to another person for support. The patient will hold a walking stick in the hand opposite the weakest leg.

If the patient has a zimmer frame, observe how he or she uses it. It is not unusual for a nervous but mobile patient to become reliant upon a frame, and on observation they will be seen to carry the frame in front of themselves, rather than rely upon it for support.

Gait

If the patient walks unaided, make a quick assessment of gait. A more formal assessment should be made later in the detailed examination.

How easily does the patient climb onto the examination couch?

A certain amount of agility is needed for elderly patients to climb onto the examination couch. It may be instructive to observe the patient during this process.

Detailed inspection

Once the patient is properly exposed and positioned, a detailed inspection should be performed. This process forms the key to a successful examination.

A detailed examination of the locomotor system is time consuming and tiring for the patient. With the benefit of the history, a focused examination is possible after detailed inspection. The more important features to note are outlined below.

Skin rash

Skin rashes may suggest:

- An underlying inflammatory illness (e.g. livedo reticularis, nailfold infarcts).
- Infection.
- Malignancy (e.g. erythema gyratum repens in breast carcinoma, dermatomyositis).
- Pain (erythema ab igne from a hot-water bottle).

Muscle bulk

Note the general muscle bulk and the distribution of any atrophy, for example:

- Disuse atrophy in a hemiplegic limb.

- Atrophy of the quadriceps in the presence of a proximal myopathy.
- Wasting of the distal muscles of the lower limbs (Charcot–Marie–Tooth disease).
- Old polio.

Deformity or swelling

Observe any obvious deformity that may be the result of bone, joint, or muscle disease, for example:

- Scoliosis.
- Varus or valgus deformity. This is common in the knees in osteoarthritis.
- Rigid back with loss of lumbar lordosis and fixed posture in ankylosing spondylitis.
- Obvious joint swelling. The distribution of swollen (or inflamed) joints should be mapped out as the distribution is often characteristic of the underlying disease and variations can be correlated with changes in disease activity (Fig. 20.1).

Gait

A formal assessment of the gait should be part of the routine examination, especially in an elderly patient. Apart from highlighting a possible aetiological factor for impaired mobility, it provides a direct functional assessment and an impression of the problems with daily living.

Ask the patient to walk in a straight line, turn around, and then walk back to you. Balance and ataxia may be additionally tested by asking the patient to walk 'heel to toe'. Observe whether the patient has any pain on walking, and if so which movements appear to provoke the pain.

Characteristic gaits may be noted as follows.

Ataxic gait

An ataxic gait is characteristically wide-based. The arms are often held out wide to aid balance. Marked clumsiness is obvious on walking heel to toe. The patient often falls to the left or right. This is associated with cerebellar pathology.

Spastic gait

If the patient has spastic paraplegia, the gait is stiff and described as a 'scissor gait'. The appearance may resemble someone wading through water. If the patient has a hemiplegia, the affected leg is extended and the leg is swung around the hip joint.

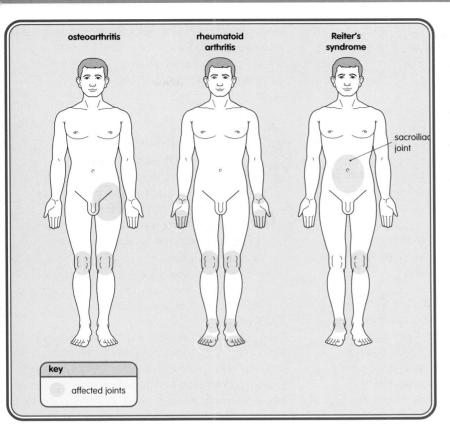

osteoarthritis   rheumatoid arthritis   Reiter's syndrome

sacroiliac joint

key

affected joints

Fig. 20.1 Typical patterns of joint involvement in three different forms of polyarthritis. In rheumatoid arthritis there is usually a symmetrical distal polyarthropathy. Osteoarthritis is less likely to be symmetrical, but often is symmetrical in its widespread form. Reiter's syndrome typically causes an asymmetrical arthropathy in the lower limbs. The hands are rarely involved.

Sensory ataxia

Peripheral neuropathy with sensory ataxia results in a gait with the appearance that the feet are being 'thrown'. The feet tend to be 'slapped' on the floor and the patient walks on a wide base. Romberg's test is positive. Patients often appear to be concentrating hard on where their feet are being placed.

High-stepping gait

In the presence of footdrop the affected foot is lifted high off the ground to avoid scraping the toes on the floor. Such patients are unable to stand on their heels.

Parkinsonian gait

The patient has a characteristic stooped appearance. The gait is shuffling and hesitant with short steps and a lack of associated arm movement. The arms are usually flexed and held at the patient's side. The gait is described as 'festinant'—having the appearance that the patient is always chasing his or her own sense of gravity. The patient often has great difficulty when asked to stop and turn around and there are usually other features of Parkinson's disease.

Osteogenic gait

Patients with legs of unequal length may walk normally in shoes with appropriate shoelifts, but the abnormality should be obvious when they walk barefoot.

Waddling gait

A proximal myopathy is associated with a waddling gait. The patient walks on a wide base with the trunk moving from side to side on each step and the pelvis drooping as the leg leaves the ground.

Regional examination

Specific regional examination can now begin. As with other systems of the body, it is important to follow a strict routine. When examining any region of the body or joint, use the following routine.

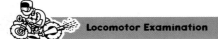
Inspection

Note the bones, alignment, joint swelling, redness, deformity, local swelling, and the presence of any scars.

Palpation

Palpate the area concerned, paying particular attention to:

- Skin temperature. In particular, note any areas of increased warmth. Compare the two sides.
- Tenderness. Map out any areas of tenderness and try to relate them to the affected structure.
- Deformity. Note the bony contours and any fixed flexion deformity.
- Soft tissues. Note the presence of any abnormal swellings (e.g cysts, bursae, tumours). Palpate the muscles for bulk and tenderness.

Assessment of joint movement

Assess the range of active and passive movement, muscular power, and whether movement is accompanied by pain. It is important to have an appreciation of the range of normal for movement around each joint. It is often helpful to test the unaffected side first so that any deviation can be more easily appreciated.

Sensation

Test the sensory modalities (see Chapter 16). Light touch, pin prick, and vibration are the most discriminatory.

Function

The most useful part of the examination is to assess the function of the relevant body part. Try to relate your assessment to daily activities, for example:

- In the lower limb test the ability to walk, jump, hop, run.
- In the hand test the ability to hold a pen and grip strength.

General examination

It is very important to perform a systemic examination. The localized joint symptoms may form part of a systemic disease or be referred from another site. Furthermore, it is possible to place the disability into context only when the patient is considered as a whole.

Some examples of this approach are given below. It is not intended to provide a detailed description of

the examination of every joint. Students are advised to refer to orthopaedic or rheumatology texts. The following examples are provided to illustrate the general approach.

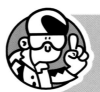

Always try to relate pathological signs to a functional disability such as difficulty in perfoming routine daily activities (e.g. getting out of bed, writing, walking, picking up a knife and fork).

Hands

Most systemic examinations start with examination of the hands, as stigmata of systemic disease are often manifest in the hands. This is also true for a patient presenting with impaired mobility. Furthermore, many patients specifically complain of symptoms directly related to their hands (e.g. paraesthesiae, weakness, joint pain). Finally, it is not uncommon for examiners to ask students to "Examine this man's hands!" A methodical approach to examination of the hands is therefore useful.

Inspection

Remember to look at the face of the patient first for any clues to the underlying disease (e.g. scleroderma, cushingoid facies). Look at both hands. Ask the patient to place his or her hands flat on the table, palmar surface downwards. Look at:

- The general shape of the hands and note any deformity (e.g. ulnar deviation in rheumatoid arthritis).
- The colour of the skin (e.g. pigmentation, icterus, erythema, rash).
- The nails. Look for signs of psoriasis (e.g. pitting, onycholysis), clubbing, splinter haemorrhages, nailfold infarcts.
- Soft tissue. Note any swellings (e.g. Heberden's nodes in osteoarthritis on the proximal and distal interphalangeal joints, gouty tophi).

- Joints. Look for any swelling or redness suggestive of an active arthritis.

Ask the patient to turn his or her hands over so that the palmar aspect can be inspected. Repeat the same process of inspection. In particular, note the presence of palmar erythema, and pay close attention to the muscle bulk of the thenar eminence (atrophy in carpal tunnel syndrome) and hypothenar eminence (atrophy in T1 root lesion or in the presence of severe rheumatoid arthritis). Note the presence of any scars (e.g. carpal tunnel decompression).

Palpation

Palpate over the joints of the hand and wrist gently, noting any tenderness. Record the distribution of any tender joints (Fig. 20.2). Many forms of polyarthritis have a characteristic distribution of joint involvement. In addition, palpate for the presence of any swellings or palmar thickening (e.g. Dupuytren's contracture, trigger finger).

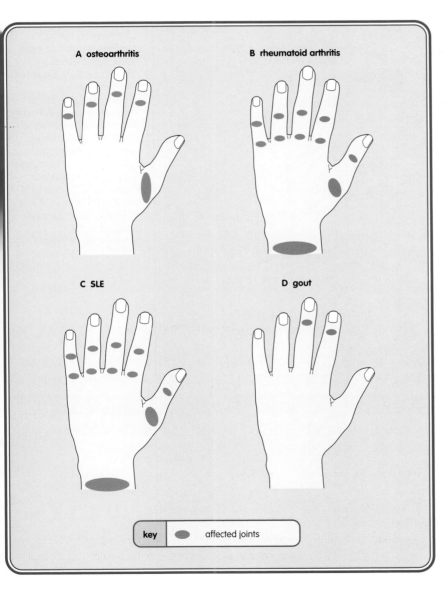

Fig. 20.2 Patterns of joint involvement in some systemic polyarthropathies. (A) Osteoarthritis (OA). Joint swelling of the first carpometacarpal joints is characteristic. Joint involvement is usually symmetrical in the hands and typically affects the distal interphalangeal joints. (B) Rheumatoid arthritis (RA). Active synovitis is detected by joint warmth, swelling, redness, and tenderness. During a flare, arthritis is usually symmetrical, affecting the wrists and metacarpophalangeal and proximal interphalangeal joints. The distal interphalangeal joints are usually spared. (C) Systemic lupus erythematosus (SLE). The distribution of joint involvement is similar to that of rheumatoid arthritis in the hands, but the signs are usually less marked and pain is often much more severe than expected from the signs of synovitis. (D) Gout. Initial attacks of gout usually present in the lower limb, especially the first metatarsophalangeal joint. However, it may present in the hands. It is often monoarticular. The distal interphalangeal joints are more prone to attacks.

Movement of the joints

Assess the movement of the joints of the hand. Try to relate this to functional activity. First, test passive movement and then active movement. If the primary problem is joint disease, useful tests might include:

- Grip strength.

- Pincer grip (ask the patient to pick up a pen and write his or her name).

Assess whether movement is limited by deformity, pain, or muscular weakness. Some of the signs of rheumatoid arthritis are illustrated in Fig. 20.3.

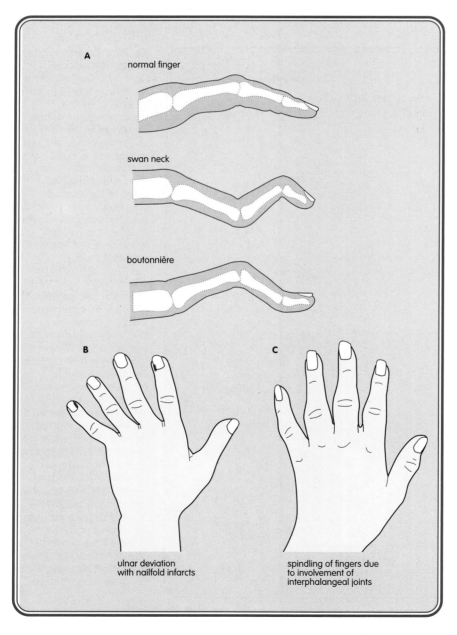

Fig. 20.3 Signs of rheumatoid arthritis in the hands. (A) Deformities of the fingers result from tendon rupture and joint laxity. Characteristic patterns include swan neck and boutonnière deformities. The thumb may develop a Z deformity. (B) Ulnar deviation results from subluxation at the metacarpophalangeal joints. Nailfold infarcts are one of the manifestations of vasculitis. (C) Spindling of the fingers is an early sign due to involvement and swelling of the interphalangeal joints.

A

normal finger

swan neck

boutonnière

B

ulnar deviation
with nailfold infarcts

C

spindling of fingers due
to involvement of
interphalangeal joints

Neurological assessment

Symptoms in the hand may result from a nerve lesion. The most common pathologies are:

- Peripheral nerve lesion (e.g. carpal tunnel syndrome, radial nerve lesion, median nerve lesion).
- Nerve root or brachial plexus lesion (e.g. Pancoast's tumour).
- Sensory neuropathy.

When examining motor and sensory function, consider the implication of each elicited physical sign and whether the underlying problem is likely to be nerve root, peripheral nerve, muscular, or joint pathology.

Motor function tests: The tests of motor function are illustrated in Fig. 20.4. If the problem is unilateral, it is very helpful to compare strength in the two hands directly, testing the normal hand first.

Sensory function tests: Test sensory function in the hand including the different modalities (pin-prick, light touch, vibration, and joint position). The distribution of sensory loss is illustrated for the three peripheral nerves, as well as the dermatomes, in Fig. 20.5. Remember that the dermatomes for the peripheral nerves or nerve roots often overlap, so it is important to test in the more discriminating areas.

Clues from the systemic examination

It should be apparent from the assessment of the hands whether the lesion is articular, vascular or neurological. There are often clues to be obtained from a systemic survey. For example:

- Look at the elbows for rheumatoid nodules or a psoriatic rash.
- Note the presence of gouty tophi on the ear lobes.

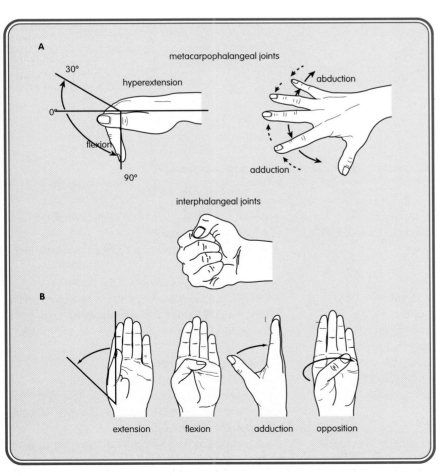

Fig. 20.4 Movements of (A) the fingers and (B) the thumb. Finger abduction and adduction (e.g. "Grip a piece of paper between your fingers!") rely on the ulnar nerve. Thumb extension relies on the radial nerve; opposition, flexion, and abduction rely on the median nerve.

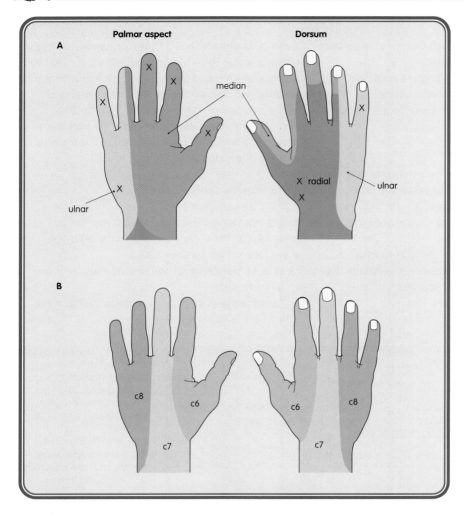

Fig. 20.5 (A) Dermatomes corresponding to the peripheral nerve supply of the hand. The crosses indicate the more useful places for assessing sensation in a quick examination.
(B) Dermatomes corresponding to the nerve root supply.

- If the patient has an arthritis, it is essential to examine each joint so that the distribution of joint involvement can be mapped out.

Back

Back pain is a very common presentation, to both general practitioners and hospital doctors. It is necessary to develop a systematic approach when examining patients with back pain so that potentially serious disease can be recognized early and investigated, while appropriate advice can be offered to the vast majority with less serious disease.

Inspection

A brief survey of the patient often provides invaluable clues. In particular, note:

- General health (e.g. cachexia suggestive of underlying malignancy).
- Posture and deformity (e.g. kyphosis, scoliosis, loss of lumbar lordosis).
- Scars (e.g. previous surgery to the back).
- Pain. Note if the patient appears to be in pain and is lying very still for fear of provoking worse pain, or if the patient appears to be comfortable and mobile.

Examination of the back

Palpate the back for heat or local tenderness suggestive of an inflammatory process. Record in the notes, the site of elicited tenderness. This may indicate the underlying disease (Fig. 20.6).

Examine the movements around the vertebrae (flexion, extension, lateral flexion, rotation) and record

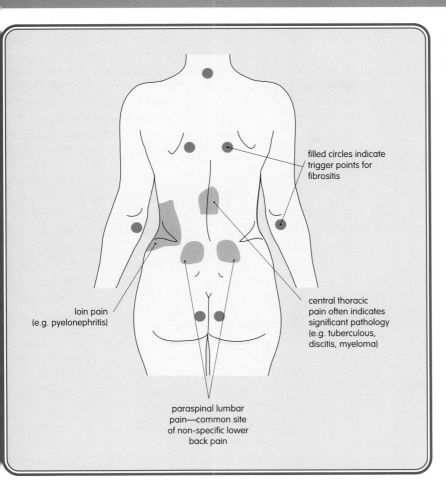

Fig. 20.6 The site of back tenderness is important as this may correspond to the aetiology.

filled circles indicate trigger points for fibrositis

central thoracic pain often indicates significant pathology (e.g. tuberculous, discitis, myeloma)

loin pain (e.g. pyelonephritis)

paraspinal lumbar pain—common site of non-specific lower back pain

both the range of movement and any pain elicited (Fig. 20.7). If ankylosing spondylitis is suspected, the sacro-iliac joints must be assessed as these are often the first site of inflammation. Lateral compression of the pelvis may elicit pain in the presence of sacro-iliitis.

Peripheral joints and systemic examination for arthritis

A full survey of other joints may reveal a more widespread arthropathy (e.g. ankylosing spondylitis, psoriatic arthropathy, Reiter's syndrome). Note the distribution of joint involvement and the presence of active synovitis.

In addition, there may also be non-articular clues to the presence of a systemic arthritis, for example:

- Psoriatic arthropathy is associated with a classical rash and nail changes.
- Ankylosing spondylitis is associated with decreased

chest expansion, upper lobe pulmonary fibrosis, iritis, and aortic regurgitation.

Test for evidence of nerve root entrapment

Acute back pain may be due to a prolapsed intervertebral disc. The presence of nerve root entrapment and its localization may be elicited by testing:

- Straight leg raising.
- Femoral stretch test (Fig. 20.8).

Neurological examination of the legs

It is important to exclude nerve root pressure or spinal cord compression. A description of the neurological assessment of the legs is given in Chapter 16, but the main points to note in the presence of back pain are:

- Muscles. Look for evidence of wasting or fasciculation. Test power. The most common sites for disc prolapse are L4–L5 (resulting in weakness of dorsiflexion and great toe extension) and L5–S1 (resulting in weakness of great toe extension).

- Sensation. Test sensation and in particular relate any sensory loss to nerve root distribution. (see Chapter 16, p. 149), assessing light touch and pin-prick sensation in the first instance (e.g. loss of sensation in the posterior and lateral aspect of the lower leg in an L4–L5 acute disc herniation). Spinal cord compression due to malignancy is often detectable by a defined 'spinal level' of sensory disturbance.

- Reflexes. Test the knee reflex (largely dependent upon L4) and the ankle reflex (largely dependent upon the S1 nerve root). If spinal cord compression is suspected the plantar response should be assessed.

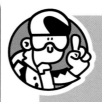

In the context of back pain, neurological examination of the legs is important. Spinal cord compression warrants urgent investigation.

Detailed systemic examination

A detailed systemic examination should always be performed in a patient presenting with new-onset or progressive back pain. The back pain may be a manifestation of a systemic disease (e.g. metastatic carcinoma) or be referred from a source in the abdomen or pelvis, for example:

- Chronic pancreatitis.
- Carcinoma of the pancreas.
- Posterior duodenal ulcer.
- Aortic aneurysm.
- Retroperitoneal fibrosis.

Hips

The hip is a common site of osteoarthritis in the elderly, but pathology sometimes begins in infancy or childhood. It is important to recognize disease early in its natural history so that appropriate treatment can be instituted.

The initial part of the examination is performed with the patient lying flat and properly exposed. Later, posture and gait can be formally assessed.

Position

Start by ensuring that the pelvis is set square so that leg length and deformity can be assessed accurately (Fig. 20.9). Attempt to position the line joining the anterior superior iliac spines perpendicular to the legs. If this is not possible, there is a fixed abduction or adduction deformity.

Fig. 20.7 Assessing movements of the (A) lumbar and (B) thoracic spine. Flexion of the lumbar spine can be measured objectively. Ask patients to touch their toes keeping their knees straight. Mark the spine at the lumbosacral junction 5 cm and 10 cm above this point. The distance between the upper two points should move approximately 5 cm on full flexion. This movement is impaired in ankylosing spondylitis.

A

10 cm
5 cm

10+ cm
5 cm

B

flexion

extension

lateral flexion

rotation

left   right

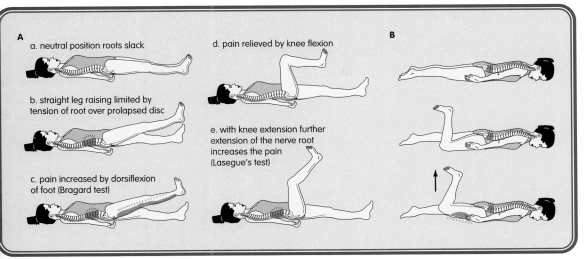

Fig. 20.8 Stretch tests. (A) Straight leg raising. Record the angle (normally 80–90 degrees) through which each leg can be raised. (B) Femoral stretch test. Ask the patient to lie on his or her front and to bend their knee. Grasp the ankle and lift the whole leg vertically upwards. Irritation of the nerve roots supplying the femoral nerve will cause pain in the anterior compartment of the thigh.

In figure A:
a. neutral position roots slack
b. straight leg raising limited by tension of root over prolapsed disc
c. pain increased by dorsiflexion of foot (Bragard test)
d. pain relieved by knee flexion
e. with knee extension further extension of the nerve root increases the pain (Lasegue's test)

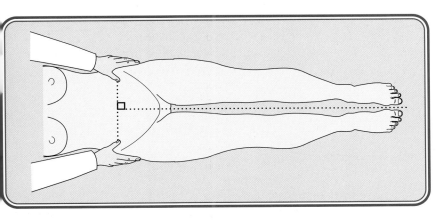

Fig. 20.9 Setting the pelvis square. Ask the patient to lie flat upon the examination couch. Palpate the anterior superior iliac spines. Move the pelvis so that the anterior superior iliac spines are square to the lower limbs.

Inspection

Note the presence of any scars (e.g. previous hip replacement), abnormal bony or soft tissue contours, and any abnormalities of the skin (e.g. erythema, sinuses).

Palpation

Palpate for any tenderness or warmth.

Measurement of leg length

If the pelvis is square, it is easy to estimate relative leg length by inspection. However, if there is any doubt, the leg can be measured from the anterior superior iliac spine to the medial malleolus (Fig. 20.10). An apparent discrepancy can be excluded by measuring the distance from the xiphisternum to the medial malleolus.

Examination for fixed deformity

Long-standing arthritis commonly results in a contracture of the joint capsule or muscles and subsequent fixed flexion deformity. Often patients compensate by increasing their lumbar lordosis (Fig. 20.11). This may be assessed by placing a hand behind the lumbar spine to detect a lordosis and then asking patients to fully flex their good leg. Push the leg further into flexion to obliterate the lordosis and observe the angle of fixed flexion deformity in the affected hip.

181

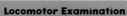

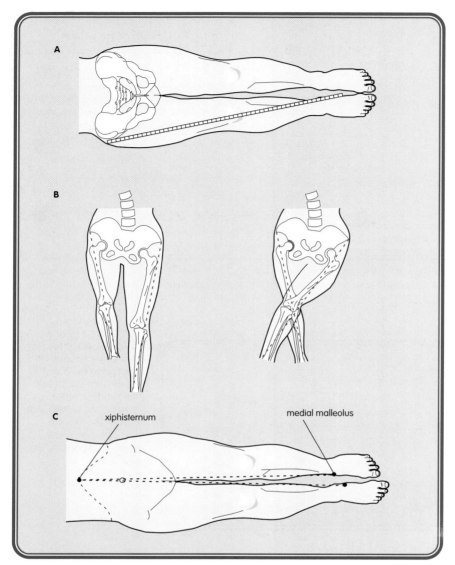

Fig. 20.10 Assessing relative leg length. (A) Measure from the anterior superior iliac spine to just below the medial malleolus on each side. (B) If the pelvis is tilted, the leg length may appear discrepant. (C) Apparent shortening may be detected measuring the distance from the xiphisternum to the medial malleolus.

A

B

C   xiphisternum   medial malleolus

Assessment of movements about the hip

It is important to assess movement about the hip and to eliminate movement of the pelvis that may compensate for deficiencies. Assess the range of movement for passive and active movements. The normal range of movement is illustrated in Fig. 20.12.

Active movement should also be tested to assess power using the Medical Research Council (MRC) grading of strength (see Fig. 16.11).

Gait and posture

Ask the patient to stand up. The Trendelenburg test should be performed to assess the postural stability of the hip joint (particularly the gluteal muscles). Normally, if one leg is lifted off the ground, the abductors will stabilize the leg and the pelvis will tilt up on the side of the lifted leg. If the abductors are ineffective, the body weight is too much for the adductors and the hip will tilt downwards (Fig. 20.13).

The causes of a positive Trendelenburg test are:
- Paralysis of the abductor muscles (e.g. polio).
- Absence of stability (e.g. ununited fracture of the femoral neck).

Finally, assess the gait.

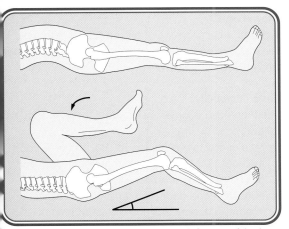

Fig. 20.11 Examination for fixed flexion deformity of the hip. A fixed deformity may be hidden by increasing the lumbar lordosis. This should be eliminated.

Normal range of movement at the hip joint	
Movement	**Range (degrees)**
flexion	0–120
extension	0 (extension occurs by rotating the pelvis)
abduction	0–30
adduction	0–30
lateral rotation	40
medial rotation	40

Fig. 20.12 Normal range of movement at the hip joint.

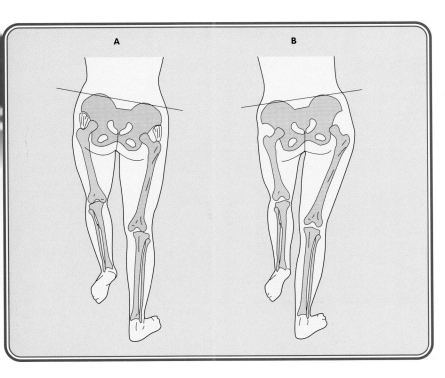

Fig. 20.13 Trendelenburg test. (A) Normally the hip abductors will tilt the pelvis upwards when the leg is lifted off the ground. (B) If the abductors cannot sustain the weight, the pelvis will droop.

Systemic survey

Remember to perform a systemic survey for other causes of the hip symptoms.

Knee

Inspection

With the patient properly exposed and supine on a couch, inspect the knee, thigh, and lower leg, noting:

- Muscle bulk and evidence of wasting.
- Bony deformity (e.g. genu varum, genu valgum, Fig. 20.14).
- Evidence of soft tissue swelling or effusion.

Palpation

Palpate the bony contours of the knee joint noting any areas of tenderness or warmth. Specifically examine for

183

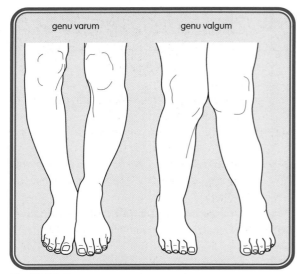

Fig. 20.14 Genu varum and genu valgum.

an effusion. A small effusion may be detectable only by massaging fluid into the suprapatellar pouch and observing accumulation in the medial compartment by pressure over the superior and lateral aspects of the joint. A larger effusion is detectable by the patellar tap.

Movements

Assess for the presence of a fixed flexion deformity, the range of passive movement, and strength of active movement.

Tests of stability

The four major ligaments should be tested in turn, as follows:

- Medial and lateral ligaments (Fig. 20.15). Support the knee in a position close to full extension and ask patients to relax their muscles. Apply an abduction and adduction force in turn to test the integrity of the medial and lateral ligaments, respectively.
- Anterior and posterior cruciate ligaments (Fig. 20.15). The anterior cruciate ligament prevents anterior displacement of the tibia on the femur; the posterior cruciate prevents posterior displacement. Flex the knee and fix the foot firmly on the couch by sitting lightly on it. Clasp the knee joint with both hands, holding your fingers behind the joint and thumbs laterally so that the tips are resting on each femoral condyle. Alternately push and pull the tibia to assess anteroposterior stability.

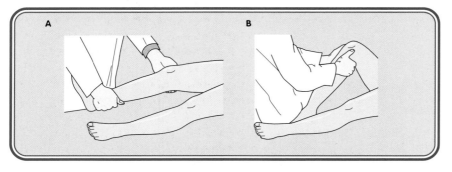

Fig. 20.15 Testing for stability of the knee joint. (A) Medial and lateral collateral ligaments. (B) Cruciate ligaments.

21. Ophthalmic Examination

Ophthalmic examination is essential in any detailed assessment of a patient. Not only may the cause of visual symptoms be determined, but the retina is the only place where the small blood vessels of the body can be directly visualized, providing clues to a host of systemic diseases.

EXAMINATION ROUTINE

Inspection

Before fundoscopy, look at the eyes for:
- Red eye (e.g. conjunctivitis, iritis, acute glaucoma, scleritis).
- Pupil size, symmetry, and irregularity.
- Pupil reflexes.
- Arcus senilis (significant in young adults).
- Squint.
- Ptosis.

Visual acuity

Test near and distant vision. Visual acuity should be tested in any complete physical examination. Test each eye individually with patients wearing their own spectacles to correct any refractive error. This need take only a few seconds, and can be adapted to different circumstances. For example:
- Read a newspaper headline from the other side of the room.
- Count fingers from the end of the bed.
- Identify light from dark, perceive hand movements.

If time permits, perform a formal assessment with a Snellen's chart (Fig. 21.1). The patient should be placed six metres from a standard chart and asked to read the letters. Each letter subtends an angle of five minutes at the defined distance (e.g. the top letter on the chart has '60' written under it, implying that it subtends this angle at a distance of 60 metres). The last line that can be clearly distinguished by the patient should be recorded for each eye. For example if the patient can read the line with '12' written under it, but not the next line, acuity in that eye is recorded as 6/12. Accepted normal vision is 6/6. The numerator refers to the distance from the chart that the patient is seated and the denominator is the last line that can be read.

Near vision can be formally tested with special books with text of a defined font and pitch size.

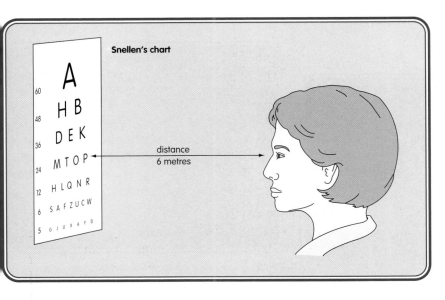

Fig. 21.1 Use of Snellen's chart to test visual acuity.

Snellen's chart

60 48 36 24 12 6 5

distance
6 metres

Eye movements and nystagmus

These are discussed in Chapter 16 (p. 137). Squint may be assessed by the cover test. If the eye fixating an object is covered, the squinting eye will move to take up fixation.

Fundoscopy

Examine in a darkened room to maximize pupil size. The patient should look straight ahead and focus on the far wall.

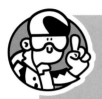

Practice fundoscopy on as many normal people as possible. It will become easier to recognise any pathological signs.

Red reflex

Start by shining the light from about 30 cm on the pupil to look for a red reflex. Loss of red reflex is usually due to vitreous haemorrhage or a dense cataract. Bring the ophthalmoscope closer to the eye and focus on the retina, looking systematically at the following.

Anterior chamber

Using a +10 lens on the ophthalmoscope, focus on the iris and examine for rubeosis or hypopyon. Then, by decreasing the power of the ophthalmoscope, focus through the anterior chamber, lens, and posterior chamber. Small cataracts appear black and well demarcated using this technique.

Optic disc

Note the size and colour of the disc. The most important pathologies to note are:

- Optic atrophy (Fig. 21.2)—may be due to multiple sclerosis, compression of the optic nerve (e.g. by pituitary tumour, aneurysm).
- Papilloedema (Fig. 21.3)—may be due to accelerated hypertension, a space-occupying lesion, hydrocephalus, benign intracranial hypertension (especially in obese women), cavernous sinus thrombosis, central retinal vein thrombosis.
- Glaucoma—pathological cupping of the disc due to gradual loss of nerve fibres and supporting glial cells, resulting in a pale disc with an enlarged cup.
- Myelinated nerve fibres.

Retina

Note the retinal vessels. Trace the vessels away from the optic disc towards each quadrant of the retina in turn. The veins are darker and appear wider than the arteries. The main features to observe about the retinal vessels are:

- Engorgement of the veins, which implies slow flow (e.g. retinal venous occlusion, polycythaemia).
- Attenuation of the arterioles (e.g. due to retinal artery occlusion, widespread retinal atrophy).
- Arteriovenous (AV) nipping in hypertension.

Note the retinal background in each quadrant. In particular, look for:
- Haemorrhages. The most common haemorrhages are flame-shaped haemorrhages, which are

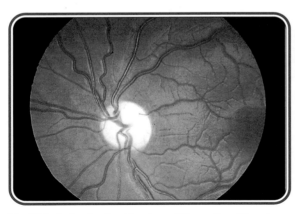

Fig. 21.2 Optic atrophy. (Courtesy of Myron Yanoff.)

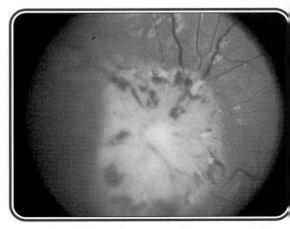

Fig. 21.3 Optic disc oedema caused by acute lymphoblastic leukaemia. (Courtesy of Myron Yanoff.)

superficial and occur in severe hypertension. 'Dot haemorrhages' are not true bleeding areas but represent microaneurysms, which are prone to rupture, forming 'blot' haemorrhages.

- Hard exudates (true retinal exudates). These are usually small, sharply defined, and intensely white.
- Soft exudates (areas of infarction). These have a fluffy appearance resembling cotton wool. They usually have an ill-defined edge.
- Neovascularization. New blood vessel formation is an important sign of diabetic retinopathy. These new blood vessels are fragile and appear as a tuft of delicate vessels on the surface of the retina.
- Photocoagulation scars.
- Pigmentation (retinitis pigmentosa).

Some of the more important fundal abnormalities are illustrated in Figs 21.4 and 21.5.

Macula

Ask the patient to look briefly directly at the light of the ophthalmoscope. Macular disease is common in the elderly.

Visual fields

The examination routine for testing by confrontation is discussed in Chapter 16 (p. 135). More formal visual field testing can be performed by assessing the visual threshold in different regions, but this relies upon special equipment and skilled interpretation.

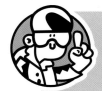

Diabetic patients should have detailed fundoscopy at least once per year.

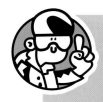

Fundoscopy provides a sensitive marker of end-organ damage in diabetes mellitus and hypertension.

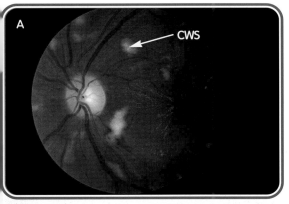

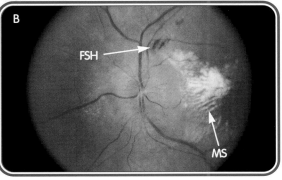

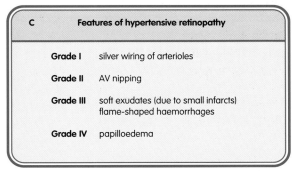

C	Features of hypertensive retinopathy
Grade I	silver wiring of arterioles
Grade II	AV nipping
Grade III	soft exudates (due to small infarcts) flame-shaped haemorrhages
Grade IV	papilloedema

Fig. 21.4 (A,B) Grade III hypertension. (CWS, cotton wool spot; FSH, flame-shaped haemorrhage; MS, Macular star.) (C) Features of hypertensive retinopathy. Grades III and IV indicate accelerated hypertension. (Courtesy of Myron Yanoff.)

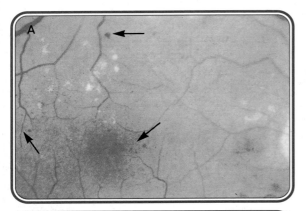

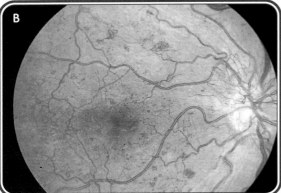

C	Features of diabetic retinopathy
Background diabetic retinopathy	
dot haemorrhages (microaneurysms)	
blot haemorrhages (discrete bleed)	
hard exudates	
Proliferative retinopathy	
neovascularization	
(laser photocoagulation scars)	

Fig. 21.5 Diabetic retinopathy. (A) Background changes (arrows point to haemorrhages). (Courtesy of Myron Yanoff.) (B) Neovascularization at the optic disc. (Courtesy of Myron Yanoff.) (C) Features of diabetic retinopathy.

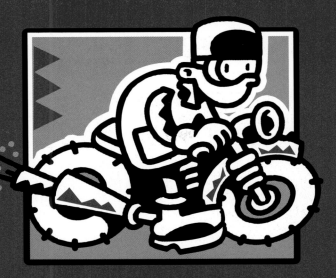

CLERKING AND FURTHER INVESTIGATIONS

22. Writing Medical Notes

GENERAL POINTS

When writing in the medical notes, it is extremely important to adopt a systematic and objective style. Your notes form a permanent record of your impression of the patient at that moment in time. It should be possible for another health care professional to read your notes and to understand them and your conclusions. Although the following points appear to be obvious, it is alarming how often simple good clinical practice is ignored. Always ensure that:

- Each piece of paper has the patient's name at its head—notes have an uncanny knack of falling apart!
- Each entry is dated and, ideally, a time recorded.
- Each entry is followed by a legible signature. Scrawled initials are inadequate. Someone else has to read your notes and be able to identify who has written them.
- Your handwriting is legible. This point sounds ludicrously obvious, but unfortunately anyone who has looked through a set of notes will testify that it is often forgotten. It is not just yourself who subsequently needs to read your notes.

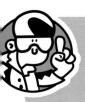

Your handwriting must be clear and legible. It is potentially dangerous to write in hieroglyphics!

- Each statement is objective. It is no longer acceptable to write value judgements in the notes if they cannot be justified. Avoid the use of meaningless phrases such as the commonly written 'This pleasant gentleman'. Does the omission of the term 'pleasant' imply that the patient is objectionable?

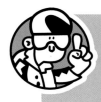

Remember that patients (or their lawyers) may gain access to the notes. Avoid the use of statements that you cannot justify.

- You write in the notes every time you see the patient. You do not have to write an essay—a short statement of the patient's progress is an important record. Even noting a lack of any change since your last consultation is important.
- You avoid the use of abbreviations as much as possible. If they have to be used, use only accepted terms such as MI (myocardial infarction), LVF (left ventricular failure).
- Facetious comments (or abbreviations) are never to be written in the notes. This goes without saying. Imagine yourself standing in court on a medical negligence claim trying to justify your statements.
- You use diagrams where appropriate as they are often much more descriptive than long paragraphs.
- You keep your record as concise as possible.

Often, the history given by the patient is recounted in an unconventional manner. When writing your notes, it is usual practice to record the history in the order described in Part I of this book. This helps to structure your own thoughts as well as those of anyone who subsequently reads the notes. Clearly, the history is a dynamic process, and there are infinite variations and exceptions to this general aim.

Finally, it is important to make a note of what information has been given to the patient. Poor communication between the doctor and patient is responsible for the vast majority of instances of patient dissatisfaction. It is helpful, not only to yourself but also for other doctors, to be aware of exactly what information the patient has been given when starting the next consultation.

STRUCTURING YOUR THOUGHTS

When you first start to take medical histories, it is a struggle to remember the traditional order of questions to ask and the normal examination routine. However, your job has only just begun! Remember that the aim of a clerking is to:

- Identify any problems.
- Formulate a differential diagnosis of these problems.
- Consider a plan of initial investigations to elucidate the underlying cause, severity, and prognosis of each problem.
- Initiate treatment and advice for the patient.

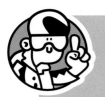

In an examination setting, it is important to spend time reflecting on the significant points of the history and examination. Always allow enough time to gather your thoughts before presenting your findings.

Once your examination has been completed, it is helpful to go through a routine and ask yourself the following questions.

What is the patient's presenting complaint?

Never forget the initial reason for the patient seeking medical attention. Although you may have identified more significant medical problems during your history and examination, you must show patients that you are addressing their primary concern.

What problems have I identified?

Problems can take many forms and be physical, social, or psychological. Before trying to dissect the differential diagnosis, it may be helpful to write down a list of each problem. A problem may be:

- A proven diagnosis (e.g. Goodpasture's syndrome).
- A pathological state (e.g. renal failure).
- An abnormal symptom (e.g. coughing up blood—haemoptysis).

- An abnormal sign (e.g. pulmonary consolidation, tachypnoea, pitting oedema).
- An abnormal investigation result (e.g. raised plasma creatinine concentration, increased carbon monoxide transfer coefficient, a raised C-reactive protein, haematuria and red cell casts in the urine).
- A past medical history (e.g. pneumonia).
- A social or psychological problem (e.g. unemployed, homelessness, intravenous drug abuser).
- Significant risk factor for illness (e.g. smoking).

It is only by identifying these individual problems and considering them as a group that their relative importance and relationship to each other can be assessed systematically.

What action is needed for each problem?

Try to prioritize the importance of each problem and decide upon the urgency of treatment and investigation of each.

What is the differential diagnosis of each problem?

By assessing each problem in turn it may become apparent that a unifying diagnosis could explain a number of features. Equally, some diagnoses may be excluded by the presence of certain features. In the example problems given above, Goodpasture's syndrome might explain the pathological state, symptoms, physical signs, and investigation results as well as the triggering of the acute illness by lung damage. However, it is also important to consider other possibilities to explain the underlying problems. For the above example, consider other causes of a pulmonary–renal syndrome such as Wegener's granulomatosis, microscopic polyangiitis, Churg–Strauss syndrome.

What is the most likely underlying diagnosis?

Once a differential diagnosis has been formulated, it is important to make a mental note of the order of probability of each diagnosis. This is important as immediate treatment and investigations are aimed at the diagnoses at the top of your list and those that require urgent therapy.

What investigations should be requested?

In the examination setting, as in real life, it is important to consider which investigations are appropriate, and their urgency. When requesting investigations it is essential to consider how the result of a particular test is going to help refine your management of the patient. It is no longer acceptable to adopt the mentality of "I always request chest radiography, an electrocardiogram, full blood count and biochemical profile for all medical patients!" Consider each problem in turn and assess which investigations are appropriate. It is by this systematic approach that potentially important and useful investigations are not omitted.

Start by considering the simple and non-invasive tests, and then consider the value of more discriminatory but invasive investigations. Weigh up the potential usefulness of the result against the potential morbidity, financial cost, (and mortality) of each test. For example:

- Many simple blood tests are cheap and non-invasive so a low threshold is needed.
- A positron emission tomograph is expensive, but in limited situations offers very specific information that cannot be obtained reliably from other sources.
- Coronary angiography is the gold standard for diagnosing structural causes of angina, but rarely results in mortality.

PRESENTING YOUR FINDINGS

It is important to get as much practice as possible in presenting your findings to your colleagues. The easiest part of a consultation is taking a history and performing an examination. Most students struggle when trying to collate the vast amount of information obtained from a clerking and to reformat it in a digestible form.

Remember how dull it can be listening to inexperienced students presenting their findings. It is essential to be as concise as possible so that important information is not lost among masses of irrelevant detail.

When presenting a clerking, put yourself in the audience's position and consider what information you would like to hear.

Start with a pithy introductory phrase describing the patient and his or her reason for presenting for medical attention. This is important as it provides a frame for the subsequent information. Your audience will already have started the process of differential diagnosis and be anticipating certain specific facts.

Describe the detailed history, using the patient's words where possible, and avoid placing value judgements at this stage. You will have asked the patient many specific questions. Your listeners are interested in a limited number of these. Using your judgement, introduce important negative responses, but do not overburden your audience with irrelevant detail. For example, if your patient presents with exertional chest pain your audience needs to know about risk factors for ischaemic heart disease and other cardiac symptoms even if there are none, but introducing information about myopia or the patient's stool habit will only cloud the important issues. The rest of the history should be presented in a similarly edited form. Unrelated symptoms described by the patient can be mentioned at the end of the history.

When presenting your examination findings:

- Start by describing the vital signs.
- Then concentrate on the system primarily affected. Discuss your findings in this system at length.
- For the other systems of the body, describe any positive findings and any important negative signs that may affect interpretation of the main findings.

It is important to sound confident. It is very difficult when you first begin, but you must commit yourself. Many students start by making excuses for having difficulty in eliciting a sign. This does not impress examiners and is not helpful—in the real world, your interpretation of physical signs affects your management of the patient.

At the end of your examination findings, provide:

- A short summary encompassing the main features of the history and examination.
- Your interpretation and analysis of the problems with a brief differential diagnosis with a note of features in favour of or against each differential diagnosis.

MEDICAL SAMPLE CLERKING

A sample medical clerking is shown below and illustrates some of the points discussed at the start of this chapter.

Details

Name:	Joe Bloggs
Date:	1st January 2000
Time:	0720h
Place:	A&E
Age:	47 years
Sex:	Male
Occupation:	HGV driver
Referred by:	Accident and Emergency Registrar

PC (presenting complaint)
4-hour crushing retrosternal chest pain

HPC (history of presenting complaint)
Onset: 4 hours of "crushing, tight" retrosternal chest pain, radiating to neck and both arms, gradual onset over 5–10 mins.
Duration: persistent since onset
Severe—"worst pain ever had"

Relieving/exacerbating factors:
GTN
provided no relief although normally relieves
pain in mins, no other relieving/exacerbating factors.

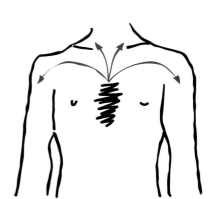

Associated symptoms:
nausea, vomiting ×2 <4>, sweating, dizzy.
1997: exertional chest tightness and dyspnoea initially controlled on atenolol.
4/12 symptoms worse, exercise tolerance 200 yards on flat, limited by chest pain.
No rest pain, no orthopnoea, no PND.

Risk factors:
Hypertension	—no.
Smoking	—20 cigarettes per day from 16 years.
FH	—father died of 'heart attack' at 53 years.
Diabetes	—no.
Cholesterol	—never checked.
Ischaemic heart disease	—angina, previous MI.

PMH (past medical history)

1963: appendectomy.
1972: duodenal ulcer (no symptoms since).
1989: gout (quiescent on treatment).
NO diabetes, hypertension, rheumatic heart disease, tuberculosis, epilepsy, asthma, jaundice, cerebrovascular disease.
1986: myocardial infarction, full recovery. No thrombolysis. No subsequent investigations.

S/E (systems enquiry)

General

Fatigue lately, appetite unchanged, weight stable, no sweats or pruritus, sleeping well.

CVS

As above.

RS

Dyspnoea on exertion, particularly uphill, but not limiting. No cough/sputum/wheeze

GIT

No current indigestion. No symptoms like previous duodenal ulcer. No vomiting/dysphagia/abdominal pain.

GUS

No urinary symptoms.

NS

No headache/syncope. No dizziness/limb weakness/sensory loss. No disturbed vision/hearing/smell/speech.

MS

No painful gout for 5 years. No joint pain/stiffness/swelling. No disability.

Skin

No rash/pruritus/bruising.

Drug history

Atenolol 100 mg once daily.
Allopurinol 300 mg nocte.
GTN as required.
Not taking aspirin.
Allergies: Penicillin: skin rash.

FH (family history)

Father died of 'heart attack' age 53.
Mother died of old age at 76.

SH (social history)
Lives with wife who is fit and well.
Own house.
Completely independent.
Smoking 20 cigs/day for many years.
Alcohol: 24 units per week.
Sexual history: not appropriate.
Overseas travel: not appropriate.
Pets: not appropriate.
Occupation: heavy goods vehicle driver.

O/E (on examination)
General:
unwell, sweaty, clammy, no cyanosis/jaundice.
Temperature: 37.5°C.
Cigarette-stained fingers.
No arcus/xanthomas/xanthelasma

CVS
Pulse 104 bpm regular, normal character.
BP 110/70 mmHg (right), 112/74 mmHg (left).
JVP normal.
No praecordial scars/chest deformities.
Apex beat displaced to anterior axillary line 6th intercostal space.
No parasternal heave/thrills.
Auscultation: Heart sounds normal, but soft pansystolic murmur at apex radiating to axilla,

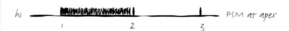

and ejection systolic murmur in aortic area with no radiation.

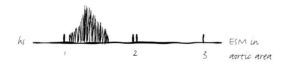

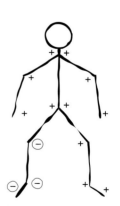

Peripheral pulses: absent right popliteal to dorsalis pedis.
No sacral or ankle oedema.

RS
Trachea central.

Respiratory rate 15/min, no respiratory distress.
Expansion symmetrical and normal.
Vocal fremitus normal.
Percussion note normal.
Breath sounds vesicular throughout, no added sounds.

Abdomen

No scars/veins/distension.
Palpation: soft, but tender LIF (left iliac fossa).
Percussion note normal.
Auscultation bowel sounds normal.
Genitalia not examined.
Rectal examination: not performed.

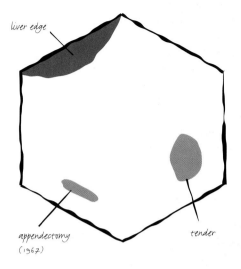

liver edge

appendectomy
(1967)

tender

NS

Higher function normal.
Cranial nerves:

    I: normal.
    II: PERRLA (pupils equal in reaction to light and accomodation)/normal fundi
    and visual fields.
    III,IV,VI: no diplopia/nystagmus.
    V: normal.
    VII: normal.
    VIII: normal.
    IX: normal.
    X: normal.
    XI: normal.
    XII: normal.

Upper and lower limbs: power, tone, coordination, sensation all normal.

Reflexes		Right	Left
	Biceps	++	++
	Supinator	++	++
	Triceps	++	++
	Knee	++	++
	Ankle	+	+
	Plantar	↓	↓

Joints and skin

Normal.

Summary

47-year-old male smoker with a family history and previous history of ischaemic heart disease, presents with a 4-month history of increasing exertional chest pain and a 4-hour history of persistent, severe pain at rest, which is unrelieved by GTN and associated with nausea, vomiting, and sweating. On examination, he has a resting tachycardia and evidence of left ventricular dilatation with a displaced apex beat and possible secondary mitral regurgitation. The most likely diagnosis is acute myocardial infarction.

Problem list

1. Chest pain ? myocardial infarction.

2. Known ischaemic heart disease—myocardial infarction, post-infarct angina.

3. Clinical left ventricular enlargement with secondary mitral regurgitation.

4. Previous duodenal ulcer but quiescent for years—no contraindications to thrombolysis.

5. Gout—can be precipitated by diuretics prescribed for cardiac failure.

6. HGV driver—should he still be driving?

The key headings to cover when taking a clerking are:
- **PC (presenting complaint)**
- **HPC (history of presenting complaint)**
- **PMH (past medical history)**
- **S/E (systems enquiry), including general, CVS, RS, GIT, GUS, NS, MS, skin**
- **Drug history**
- **Allergies**
- **FH (family history)**
- **SH (social history)**
- **O/E (on examination), including general, CVS, RS, abdomen, NS, reflexes**
- **Joints and skin**
- **Summary**
- **Problem list**

23. Further Investigations

Once the history and examination have been performed, it is necessary to assess your differential diagnosis and to plan a management strategy for the patient. Part of this process includes arranging further investigations in order to refine the differential diagnosis. The tests may be performed to:
- Exclude serious conditions.
- Confirm the presence of a suspected pathology.
- Obtain a baseline against which further progress may be assessed.
- Assess the severity of the current illness.
- Assess the response to therapy.
- Predict prognosis.

Remember that it is easy to request investigations, but the results may require great skill in interpretation. Furthermore, each test has a cost and produces a defined morbidity (however small) to the patient. It is essential to anticipate how the results of the investigation may alter your management at the time of the request. If you cannot see how the results of an investigation will alter your management, there is absolutely no point in requesting that test. For each test, justify:
- Why it is being requested.
- How the result will affect management.
- That the potential benefit of the information outweighs the cost and morbidity incurred.
- The urgency of a request.

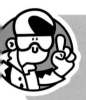

Before requesting any investigation think how the patient will benefit from the result.

The lists given below are not intended to be comprehensive, and certainly do not imply that every test should be requested for each system. The tests requested need to be tailored to the clinical scenario. For each system, consider:
- Blood.
- Urine.

- Radiological imaging.
- Electrical recording.
- Special investigations.

CARDIOVASCULAR SYSTEM

Blood tests

The following blood tests may help in the diagnosis of cardiac pathologies:
- Full blood count. Anaemia may be the cause of or exacerbate heart failure or angina.
- Erythrocyte sedimentation rate (ESR). Inflammatory conditions (e.g. endocarditis) are associated with a raised ESR. The C-reactive protein (CRP) is an acute phase protein and is often more sensitive than the ESR in changing inflammatory states (e.g. monitoring the response of infective endocarditis to antibiotic therapy).
- Cardiac enzymes. Muscle necrosis in myocarditis or myocardial infarction will produce an elevated level of creatine kinase (CK), aspartate transaminase (AST), and lactate dehydrogenase (LDH) after a characteristic time point (Fig. 23.1).
- Biochemical profile. Exclude electrolyte disturbance as a cause of arrhythmia.

The diagnosis of acute myacardial infarction is made on the history and characteristic ECG changes. Blood tests usually provide retrospective confirmation.

- Thyroid function tests. Hyperthyroidism is a common cause of atrial fibrillation. Hypothyroidism may present as a pleural effusion or heart failure.
- Blood cultures. Essential if endocarditis is suspected.
- Protein C, S, factor V Leiden, antithrombin III, lupus anticoagulant. Request for idiopathic thromboembolic disease.

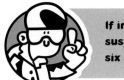

If **infective endocarditis is suspected obtain at least six sets of blood culture.**

• Signs of left atrial enlargement—prominence of atrial appendage (straight left heart border), double contour of right heart border, splaying of the carina.
• Left ventricular aneurysm—post-myocardial infarction.
• Abnormal calcification—valvular calcification in rheumatic heart disease, tuberculous pericardial disease (Fig. 23.3).

Echocardiography

Echocardiography may be transthoracic (non-invasive) or transoesophageal, which provides better images of the left atrium and aorta. It is useful for assessing chamber size, valvular pathology, pericardial disease, and contractility of the heart. Echocardiography is usually requested to:

• Exclude treatable causes of heart failure.
• Investigate heart murmurs.
• Look for vegetations in suspected infective endocarditis.
• Investigate pericardial effusions and tamponade.
• Assess the severity of cor pulmonale.
• Investigate aortic aneurysms.

Modifications of echocardiography, such as stress echo and contrast echo, may also be used to investigate angina and septal defects, respectively. The two most common views are illustrated in Figs 23.4 and 23.5.

Nuclear imaging

Nuclear imaging (e.g. thallium scan) can be used to investigate suspected angina in a patient who cannot perform an exercise test.

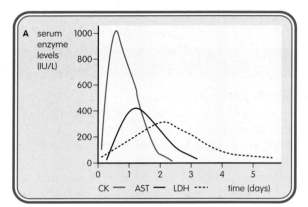

B	Change in the 'cardiac enzymes' with time following a myocardial infarction		
Enzyme	Time to start rise (h)	Time to peak elevation (h)	Duration of elevation (days)
CK	4–6	24–48	3–5
AST	8–12	24–48	4–6
LDH	24	48–72	7–10

Fig. 23.1 (A) Graph and (B) table to show the change in the 'cardiac enzymes' with time following a myocardial infarction. (AST, aspartate transaminase; CK, creatine kinase; LDH, lactate dehydrogenase.)

Urinalysis

Look for microscopic haematuria if infective endocarditis is suspected.

Imaging
Chest radiography

A chest radiograph is usually requested for a patient who presents with cardiological symptoms. Note the presence of:

• Cardiac enlargement—cardiothoracic ratio should be less than 50% (posteroanterior film).
• Signs of increased left atrial filling pressure—upper lobe blood diversion, septal lines, pulmonary oedema, pleural effusion (Fig. 23.2).

Electrocardiography (ECG)
12-lead ECG

ECGs are very widely performed. They can be used to assess wide-ranging cardiac pathologies such as rhythm disturbances, ischaemia or infarction, left ventricular hypertrophy, right ventricular hypertrophy.

24-hour tape (Holter monitor)

A 24-hour tape is used to investigate paroxysmal cardiac arrhythmias that may be associated with symptoms. Patients should be instructed to indicate when they have palpitations or other symptoms such as lightheadedness so that their symptoms can be correlated with electrical disturbances.

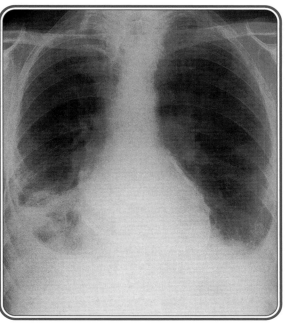

Fig. 23.2 Radiograph of left heart failure. Note the cardiomegaly, bilateral alveolar shadowing in a perihilar distribution, and the presence of fluid in the horizontal fissure.

Fig. 23.3 Radiograph of pericardial calcification. Note the associated pleural effusions.

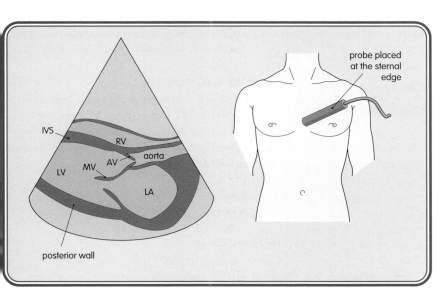

Fig. 23.4 Diagrammatic representation of a normal parastemal view of the left ventricle. The probe is placed in the left parasternal region. This provides a good view for assessing chamber size, left ventricular wall motion, and ejection fraction, as well as mitral and aortic valve regurgitation using colour Doppler. (AV, aortic valve; IVS, interventricular septum; LA, left atrium; LV, left ventricle; MV, mitral valve; RV, right ventricle.)

Event recorder (cardiac memo)

If the palpitation lasts long enough, it is desirable to record the ECG at the time of the arrhythmia. Symptoms can then be directly related to the electrical activity of the heart.

Exercise ECG

The exercise ECG is used as a screening test in the investigation of ischaemia. Many cardiologists do not refer patients for angiography if the exercise test is

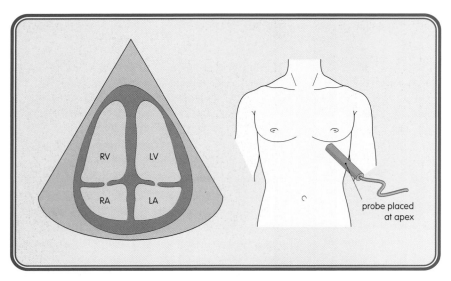

Fig. 23.5 Diagrammatic representation of a four-chamber view. The probe is placed at the apex. This view allows assessment of the left ventricular apex and quantification of the severity of aortic and tricuspid valve pathology. (LA, left atrium; LV, left ventricle; RA, right atrium; RV, right ventricle.)

normal. In addition, exercise testing provides collateral information on exercise tolerance. Remember that it is a waste of time requesting an exercise test for a wheelchair-bound 90-year-old!

Coronary angiography
This invasive investigation is used:
- To assess the coronary arteries.
- To measure pressures in the heart chambers and great vessels in the assessment of valve pathology or cor pulmonale.

RESPIRATORY SYSTEM

Blood tests
Patients with respiratory disease often have infections or unexplained dyspnoea. The more common blood tests requested include:
- Full blood count. A raised white cell count suggests infection. A raised eosinophil count may occur in rare conditions such as pulmonary eosinophilic syndrome and Churg–Strauss syndrome, and atopic conditions.
- ESR—raised during active inflammatory states.
- Blood cultures—important in the diagnosis of pneumonia.
- Viral, *Mycoplasma*, *Legionella*, chlamydial serology—used in the diagnosis of pneumonia.
- Arterial blood gases—essential in the assessment of severe asthma attacks and for providing baseline

function for patients with chronic obstructive pulmonary disease (COPD).

Perform serological tests in the acute and convalescent phase of the illness. A four-fold rise in titre usually confirms the underlying diagnosis

Sputum assessment
Sputum culture is part of the routine assessment of a patient with a chest infection. When investigating pneumonia, especially in sick patients, liaison with the laboratory is important for diagnosing some of the less common infections (e.g. *Pneumocystis*, mycobacteria, *Nocardia*).

Sputum cytology is used in the investigation of malignancy and certain pneumonias.

Imaging
Chest radiography
In the context of respiratory disease, the important features to note are:
- Area of consolidation—for example lobar, widespread.
- Evidence of COPD—paucity of lung vascular markings, hyperinflation, flat diaphragms, narrow mediastinum, bullae.

- Pneumothorax or areas of collapse in asthmatic patients.
- Hilar masses—lung carcinoma may underlie many respiratory disorders (Fig. 23.6); bilateral lymphadenopathy occurs in sarcoidosis.
- Pleural effusions.
- Fibrosis.

Computerized tomography (CT) scan

Occasionally CT scanning is needed to clarify features on the radiograph, for example:

- Investigation of direct or metastatic spread of suspected lung cancer.
- Investigation of bronchiectasis.
- Investigation of pulmonary fibrosis.

Lung function tests

Assessment of gas exchange and airway function may be performed by the following methods.

Peak expiratory flow rate

This should be considered as part of the routine examination of the asthmatic patient.

Arterial blood gases

These are useful for assessing gas exchange in acute pulmonary disease. In addition they provide a baseline assessment for patients with COPD when they are stable (e.g. on discharge from hospital).

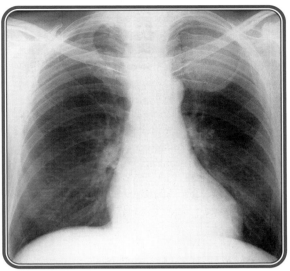

Fig. 23.6 Radiograph of a Pancoast tumour with destruction of the first left rib.

Spirometry

The most simple assessments of forced expiratory volume in one second (FEV_1) and forced vital capacity (FVC) can provide invaluable information in respiratory disease. The ratio of FEV_1/FVC and absolute values will help in the diagnosis of:

- Obstructive disease—low ratio (< 70%) and low absolute values.
- Restrictive disease—normal or high ratio, reduced FVC (Fig. 23.7).

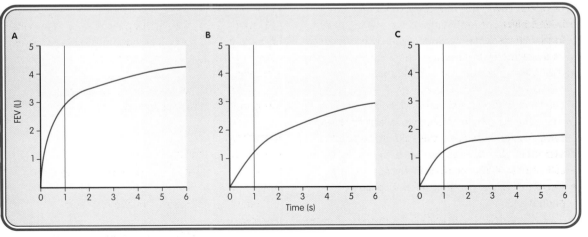

Fig. 23.7 Examples of spirometry. (A) Normal patient—FEV_1/FVC = 3.0/4.0 (75%). (B) chronic obstructive pulmonary disease—FEV_1/FVC = 1.5/3.0 (50%). (C) Fibrosis—FEV_1/FVC = 1.5/1.8 (83%).

In addition, the absolute value of FEV_1 is often used to assess patients with respiratory muscle weakness (e.g. myasthenia gravis, Guillain–Barré syndrome).

Variations can be used to record bronchial reactivity to allergens or potential reversibility with bronchodilators.

The transfer coefficient of carbon monoxide (K_{CO}) provides a measure of the efficiency of gas exchange and permeability of the alveolar membrane:
- Diseases resulting in impaired ventilation or perfusion reduce K_{CO}.
- Diseases such as pulmonary haemorrhage increase K_{CO}.

Bronchoscopy

Bronchoscopy allows direct visualization of the upper airways and abnormal areas can be biopsied. In addition, bronchoalveolar lavage can be performed to collect specimens for culture and cytology and to assess the different cell types in the alveoli.

ABDOMINAL SYSTEM

Blood tests

Blood tests are required for a wide range of abdominal presentations including the investigation of anaemia, jaundice, palpable masses, abdominal pain, and bowel disturbance.

The more commonly requested investigations include:
- Full blood count. This may reveal anaemia. The mean cell volume (MCV) provides a starting point for further investigation. A raised white count suggests an inflammatory process.
- ESR. Raises the suspicion of inflammatory lesions, if raised.
- Biochemical profile. Assess liver function, renal function, and calcium. Electrolyte levels may fluctuate during diarrhoeal illnesses or fluid replacement.
- Vitamin B_{12}, iron studies, red cell folate levels. These are initial investigations in anaemia.
- Amylase. Exclude pancreatitis as a cause of abdominal pain.

Urinalysis

Urinalysis is part of the routine assessment during a detailed examination. Note the presence of:

- Glycosuria—diabetes mellitus.
- Haematuria—for example due to glomerulonephritis, renal stone, bladder lesion.
- Proteinuria.
- Ketonuria—diabetic ketoacidosis.
- Nitrites or leucocytes—indicate infection.

Imaging
Chest radiography
An erect chest radiograph is often requested for patients presenting with acute abdominal pain. The important features to note are:
- The presence of free air under the diaphragm—suggests perforated viscus (Fig. 23.8).
- Lower lobe consolidation—pneumonia masquerading as acute abdominal pain.

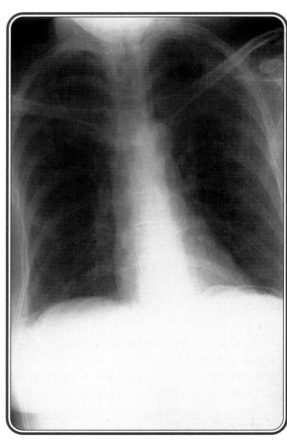

Fig. 23.8 Air under the diaphragm. This suggests the presence of a perforated abdominal viscus.

Abdominal radiography

The main features to note are:

- Distended loops of bowel—suggestive of bowel obstruction.
- Double contour to the bowel—perforation with free air in the abdomen (Wriggler's sign).
- Radio-opaque gallstones—unusual (only 10%).
- Radio-opaque renal calculi—common (i.e. 90%).

Abdominal ultrasound and CT scan

These are performed to localize and identify any abnormal masses, detect free fluid in the abdomen, and assess the size and parenchyma of intra-abdominal organs.

Ultrasound is particularly useful in the assessment of jaundice as biliary tree dilatation and gallstones are readily identified.

Following trauma, CT or ultrasound may be used to diagnose damage to the liver, kidney, or spleen.

Barium studies

Barium studies are used to assess abnormalities of the mucosa or motility disorders. The four main studies are:

- Barium swallow—to assess the oesophagus (e.g. for dysphagia, heartburn).
- Barium meal—to assess mucosal abnormalities of the stomach and duodenum (e.g. for dyspepsia, iron-deficiency anaemia).
- Small-bowel meal or enema—to assess the small bowel, in particular the terminal ileum (e.g. for malabsorption, suspected Crohn's disease).
- Barium enema—to investigate the colon (e.g. for anaemia, change in bowel habit, rectal bleeding).

Endoscopy

Endoscopy is performed to visualize the mucosa of the bowel directly and to biopsy any abnormal area. Upper gastrointestinal (GI) endoscopy will assess as far as the duodenum. A good colonoscopy will reveal the whole of the large bowel.

Endoscopic retrograde cholangiopancreatography (ERCP) can be performed to image the pancreatic or hepatic and bile ducts and to treat any strictures or remove stones.

Stool assessment

Stool assessment may involve:

- Culture—diarrhoeal illnesses.
- Microscopy—for ova, cysts and parasites.
- Faecal fat estimation.
- Occult blood test.

RENAL SYSTEM

Blood tests

A diagnosis of renal failure is largely dependent upon laboratory investigations. Many of these tests require experience in interpretation. A daunting list of investigations is given below, but the specific mode of presentation must be taken into account to determine which are appropriate:

- Full blood count and blood film.
- ESR—it is often raised in renal failure of any cause.
- CRP—better marker of inflammation in renal disease than ESR.
- Biochemical profile—for renal function, acid–base status, electrolyte disturbances, liver function, calcium, phosphate.
- Glucose.
- Blood cultures.
- Protein electrophoresis—especially if possible myeloma or cryoglobulinaemia.
- Autoantibodies.
- Complement levels
- Serology for systemic lupus erythematosus (SLE) and rheumatoid arthritis.
- Cryoglobulins.
- Antineutrophil cytoplasmic antibody (ANCA)—vasculitis.
- Antiglomerular basement membrane antibody—Goodpasture's disease.
- Hepatitis B and C serology.
- HIV serology—remember that proper counselling and consent are essential.

Urinalysis

Urine dipstick analysis should be performed for blood and protein. A centrifuged fresh sample should be analysed under the microscope in acute renal failure for the presence of casts or red cells, which may suggest glomerulonephritis.

Urinary electrolytes may occasionally be useful, for example in the diagnosis of prerenal disease or hepatorenal syndrome.

24-hour urine collections are often made to estimate

glomerular filtration rate (GFR), protein excretion, or the excretion of certain electrolytes.

Imaging
Renal ultrasound scan
The main purpose of a renal ultrasound scan in acute renal failure is to:
- Assess renal size (e.g. to determine whether the kidney is large enough to biopsy, look for asymmetry).
- Exclude hydronephrosis.

Renal CT scan
CT scans are used to assess renal masses or to investigate trauma.

Nuclear medicine scans
Nuclear medicine images provide:
- Data about the relative GFR of the kidneys.
- Evidence of renal scarring.
- Information on possible obstruction to outflow.

Intravenous pyelography (IVP)
IVP provides detailed information on renal anatomy and the presence of renal stones (Fig. 23.9). It is often requested for investigation of haematuria to assess the collecting system and ureters.

Renal biopsy
In many cases of renal failure due to suspected glomerulonephritis, the only way of obtaining an accurate diagnosis is by performing a percutaneous renal biopsy under local anaesthetic.

NEUROLOGICAL SYSTEM

Imaging
CT scans and magnetic resonance imaging (MRI) of the brain or spinal cord are often requested to investigate acute and chronic neurological symptoms. CT is the modality of choice in the investigation of acute trauma or subarachnoid haemorrhage.

Electroencephalography (EEG)
The EEG relates to the brain in the same way that the ECG relates to the heart. However, correlation between the traces and physiological function is less understood.

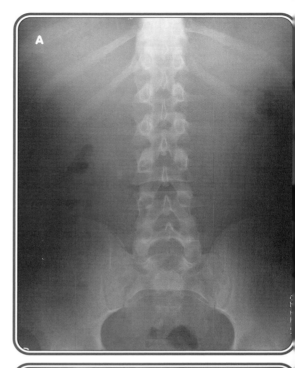

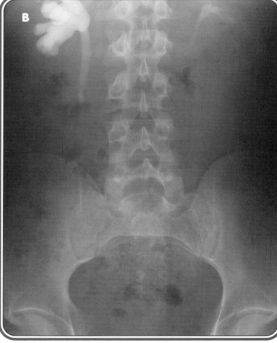

Fig. 23.9 Intravenous pyelography. (A) Control (pre-contrast image) showing the presence of calcification to the right of L3. (B) After administration of contrast, the left collecting system appears normal, but there is obvious dilatation of the right collecting system and ureter to the level of the stone.

The main uses of the EEG are in:
- Diagnosis of epilepsy.
- Diagnosis of encephalitis.

Lumbar puncture

Lumbar puncture provides essential information in the assessment of patients with neurological disease, especially those with suspected meningitis. The main indications are:
- Investigation of meningitis.
- Pyrexia of unknown origin.
- Subarachnoid haemorrhage.

In the presence of decreased level of consciousness or focal neurological signs, obtain a CT scan of the brain before performing a lumbar puncture.

- Inflammatory central nervous system (CNS) disease (e.g. multiple sclerosis, vasculitis).

Lumbar puncture is contraindicated in the presence of:
- Suppuration of the skin overlying the spinal canal.
- Undiagnosed papilloedema.

Electromyography (EMG)

EMG is used in the assessment of the peripheral nervous system. It is particularly useful if the patient reports:
- Weakness or wasting.
- Undue fatiguability.
- Sensory impairment or paraesthesia.

EMG will establish a diagnosis of a neuropathy and identify the pathological process as a demyelination or axonal neuropathy. In addition, diagnostic information may be provided for some myopathies.

Evoked potentials

Visual evoked potentials are sometimes used in the assessment of a patient with suspected multiple sclerosis.

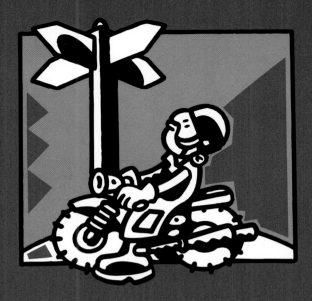

SELF-ASSESSMENT

Multiple-choice Questions

Indicate whether each answer is true or false.

1. When assessing cardiac murmurs:

a) The loudness of the murmur correlates with the severity of aortic stenosis.
b) The presence of a presystolic accentuation of the murmur of mitral stenosis indicates a tight stenosis.
c) The length of the murmur of mitral stenosis correlates with the severity of the valve disease.
d) The murmur of aortic regurgitation is most easily heard using the bell of the stethoscope.
e) Aortic stenosis is associated with a 'tapping' apex beat.

2. Following a myocardial infarction:

a) A long systolic murmur is characteristic of mitral valve papillary muscle rupture.
b) Bradycardia is more common following an inferior myocardial infarction.
c) In the acute setting, atrial fibrillation occurs in approximately 10% of patients.
d) In the acute setting, heart failure is usually detected by the presence of pitting oedema of the ankles.
e) Left ventricular aneurysm is a late complication.

3. When assessing a patient with unilateral chest disease:

(a) The side with reduced expansion always indicates the side of the pathology.
(b) The trachea deviates towards the side of the pathology.
(c) Lobar consolidation is readily distinguished from pulmonary fibrosis by the quality of the crackles.
(d) A unilateral pleural effusion is due to an exudate.
(e) The loudness of the wheezes correlates with the severity of an acute asthmatic attack.

4. In a patient presenting with a pneumonic illness:

(a) If the patient owns a parrot, the most likely responsible agent for a community-acquired pneumonia is *Chlamydia psittaci*.
(b) A history of exposure to farm animals is relevant for possible infection with *Nocardia asteroides*.
(c) Herpes labialis is a recognized association of pneumococcal pneumonia.
(d) Transplant recipients are particularly susceptible to infection with cytomegalovirus.
(e) Gram-negative infections are more common in hospitalized patients.

5. In a jaundiced patient:

(a) Hepatitis C usually presents as a fulminant hepatic illness.
(b) A history of drug abuse is relevant for hepatitis A infection.
(c) Recent ingestion of primaquine may provoke a haemolytic crisis in glucose-6-phosphate dehydrogenase deficiency.
(d) A history of pruritus suggests obstructive jaundice.
(e) The most common cause of jaundice in hospitalized patients is a drug reaction.

6. In a diabetic patient with chronic renal failure:

(a) In the presence of retinopathy and neuropathy, the cause of renal failure is most likely to be diabetic glomerulosclerosis.
(b) Angiotensin-converting enzyme (ACE) inhibitors should be used with caution if there is a history of claudication.
(c) Nephrotic-range proteinuria makes a diagnosis of diabetic glomerulosclerosis unlikely.
(d) The presence of microscopic haematuria makes diabetic glomerulosclerosis less likely.
(e) Anaemia is common.

211

7. **Risk factors for a fatal drug overdose include:**

(a) Old age.
(b) Male sex.
(c) Underlying medical illness.
(d) Alcohol abuse.
(e) Ingestion of temazepam.

8. **Features in the history to suggest a potentially serious underlying cause for a headache include:**

(a) Sudden onset.
(b) Presence of a prodrome.
(c) Scalp tenderness.
(d) Late-evening headache.
(e) Neck stiffness.

9. **In a patient presenting with back pain:**

(a) Thoracic pain is likely to represent significant organic disease.
(b) Depression is common.
(c) Psoriasis is associated with spondylosis.
(d) A positive femoral stretch test is associated with disc prolapse of the L2–L3 disc.
(e) Abdominal examination is essential.

10. **In a patient with rheumatoid arthritis treated with gold injections, side effects include:**

(a) Hepatotoxicity.
(b) Skin rash.
(c) Stomatitis.
(d) Retinopathy.
(e) Proteinuria.

11. **Presenting features of thyrotoxicosis include:**

(a) Palpitations.
(b) Constipation.
(c) Poor concentration.
(d) Cold intolerance.
(e) Pretibial myxoedema.

12. **Lesions of the visual pathway typically produce the following visual field defects:**

(a) Expanding pituitary tumour—homonymous hemianopia.
(b) Optic neuritis—homonymous hemianopia.
(c) Lesion of the optic tract—homonymous hemianopia.
(d) Lesion of the optic radiation in the left parietal lobe—upper right quadrantic hemianopia.
(e) Lesion of the optic radiation in the right temporal lobe—upper left quadrantic hemianopia.

13. **In the lower limb:**

(a) Innervation of the ankle jerk is from S1–S2.
(b) Eversion of the foot is derived from S1.
(c) Hip extension is derived from L2–L3.
(d) The cremasteric reflex is derived from S1.
(e) Knee extension is derived from L2–L4.

14. **The following typically cause massive splenomegaly:**

(a) Portal hypertension.
(b) Chronic myeloid leukaemia.
(c) Myelofibrosis.
(d) Chronic lymphatic leukaemia.
(e) Subacute infective endocarditis.

15. **Nailfold infarcts and peripheral neuropathy are associated with:**

(a) Systemic lupus erythematosus (SLE).
(b) Diabetes mellitus.
(c) Mixed essential cryoglobulinaemia.
(d) Charcot–Marie–Tooth syndrome.
(e) Wegener's granulomatosis.

16. **Features of a unilateral upper motor neuron (UMN) lesion include:**

(a) Flaccid paralysis.
(b) Brisk reflexes.
(c) Sparing of the upper half of the face in facial muscle weakness.
(d) Decreased sensation in the perineal region.
(e) Clasp-knife rigidity.

17. The lymphatic drainage of the following organs is as follows:

a) Breast—axilla.
b) Testis—inguinal.
c) Stomach—left supraclavicular.
d) Kidney—para-aortic.
e) Skin of the penis—inguinal.

18. Features very suggestive of malignancy during examination of the breast include:

a) Peau d'orange.
b) A mobile lump.
c) Palpable axillary lymphadenopathy.
d) Tenderness of the breast.
e) Retraction of the nipple.

19. Causes of optic atrophy include:

a) Multiple sclerosis.
b) Glaucoma.
c) Toxic amblyopia.
d) Cavernous sinus thrombosis.
e) Friedreich's ataxia.

20. Rheumatoid arthritis:

a) Characteristically produces a symmetrical distal polyarthropathy.
b) Is associated with vasculitis.
c) Usually involves the proximal and distal interphalangeal joints.
d) Is associated with amyloidosis of the kidneys.
e) Is associated with psoriasis.

21. The following conditions are commonly associated with atrial fibrillation:

a) Mitral stenosis.
b) Congenital lymphoedema.
c) Hypothyroidism.
d) Opiate overdose.
e) Amphetamine overdose.

22. A pleural effusion associated with the following conditions is usually an exudate:

(a) Nephrotic syndrome due to focal segmental glomerulosclerosis.
(b) Hypothyroidism.
(c) Ovarian fibroma.
(d) Rheumatoid arthritis.
(e) Pancreatitis.

23. Lung fibrosis is associated with exposure to:

(a) Busulphan.
(b) Asbestos.
(c) Cimetidine.
(d) Beryllium.
(e) Pigeons.

24. The following occupations and conditions are associated with each other:

(a) Animal laboratory technician—extrinsic allergic alveolitis.
(b) Farmers—leptospirosis.
(c) Health care workers—hepatitis B.
(d) Abattoir workers—cytomegalovirus pneumonia.
(e) Unemployment—suicide.

25. The following physical signs may be detected in anaemic patients:

(a) Koilonychia in a patient with folate deficiency.
(b) A beefy red sore tongue in a patient with vitamin B_{12} deficiency.
(c) Angular stomatitis in a patient with folate deficiency.
(d) Mild jaundice in a patient with haemolytic anaemia.
(e) Bossing of the skull in a patient with thalassaemia major.

26. Blue sclerae are a recognized association with:

(a) Rheumatoid arthritis.
(b) Psoriatic arthritis.
(c) Osteogenesis imperfecta.
(d) Rickets.
(e) Diabetes mellitus.

27. Carpal tunnel syndrome:

(a) Characteristically results in wasting of the hypothenar eminence.
(b) Is associated with pregnancy.
(c) Is associated with rheumatoid arthritis.
(d) Causes sensory loss in the palmar aspect of the radial three and a half digits.
(e) Produces sensory signs in the C5 dermatome.

28. Symptoms of uraemia include:

(a) Anorexia.
(b) Muscle twitching.
(c) Confusion.
(d) Hiccough.
(e) Hyperventilation.

29. Polycystic kidney disease in adults:

(a) Is the most common cause of bilateral palpable kidneys.
(b) Is inherited in an autosomal dominant manner.
(c) Is associated with hypertension.
(d) Is usually associated with tenderness of the kidneys on palpation.
(e) May present with haematuria.

30. Polycythaemia is associated with:

(a) Splenomegaly.
(b) Heavy smoking.
(c) Polycystic ovaries.
(d) Cerebellar haemangioblastoma.
(e) Hepatocellular carcinoma.

31. Side effects of long-term glucocorticosteroid use include:

(a) Osteomalacia.
(b) Proximal myopathy.
(c) Adrenal suppression.
(d) Diabetes insipidus.
(e) Cataracts.

32. Stigmata of chronic liver disease include:

(a) Beau's lines.
(b) Necrobiosis lipoidica.
(c) Small testicles.
(d) Scanty axillary hair.
(e) Erythema nodosum.

33. Vitiligo is associated with:

(a) Hypothyroidism.
(b) Osteomalacia.
(c) Cerebellar haemangioblastoma.
(d) Folate deficiency.
(e) Diabetes mellitus.

34. The following are associated with malignancy:

(a) Erythema gyratum repens.
(b) Lupus pernio.
(c) Ichthyosis.
(d) Erythema chronicum migrans.
(e) Tylosis.

35. The following statements regarding psoriasis are correct:

(a) Classic plaque psoriasis typically affects the flexor surfaces.
(b) Guttate psoriasis is more common in the elderly.
(c) Erythrodermic psoriasis is a cause of high-output cardiac failure.
(d) Psoriatic arthropathy is associated with nail changes of psoriasis.
(e) It may be exacerbated by β-blockers.

36. Signs of cerebellar dysfunction include:

(a) Increased muscle tone.
(b) Exaggerated tendon reflexes.
(c) Resting tremor.
(d) Unsteady gait.
(e) Dysarthria characterized by jerky speech.

37. With regard to the tendon reflexes:

a) The peripheral nerve supply of the biceps reflex is the ulnar nerve.
b) The peripheral nerve supply of the brachioradialis reflex is the radial nerve.
c) The peripheral nerve supply of the triceps reflex is the median nerve.
d) The peripheral nerve supply of the knee reflex is the femoral nerve.
e) The nerve roots supplying innervation to the supinator reflex are C8–T1.

38. The following statements with regard to the extraocular muscles are correct:

a) The inferior oblique is innervated by the oculomotor nerve.
b) A IVth nerve lesion results in inability to look down when the eye is adducted.
c) A IIIrd nerve palsy results in an eye that is abducted and looking downwards.
d) A VIth nerve palsy is always due to a lesion in the pons.
e) Superior rectus elevates the eye.

39. With regard to hernias:

a) The femoral hernia is the most common abdominal hernia in women.
b) A direct inguinal hernia often descends into the scrotum.
c) The origin of a femoral hernia is below and medial to the pubic tubercle.
d) Para-umbilical hernias are more common than true umbilical hernias.
e) Pregnancy is a risk factor.

40. Risk factors for pancreatitis include:

a) Oxalosis.
b) Gallstones.
c) Primary hypercalciuria.
d) Azathioprine.
e) Doxazosin.

41. With regard to peptic ulceration:

(a) Gastric and duodenal ulceration can usually be reliably differentiated from the history.
(b) It may present with back pain.
(c) It is associated with cigarette smoking.
(d) It is more common in women.
(e) A past history of peptic ulcer is an absolute contraindication to thrombolysis.

42. The following diseases are more common in women:

(a) Hyperthyroidism.
(b) Femoral hernia.
(c) Primary biliary cirrhosis.
(d) Systemic lupus erythematosus.
(e) Motor neuron disease.

43. The following conditions typically present with red urine:

(a) Horseshoe kidney.
(b) Excessive beetroot consumption.
(c) Nephrotic syndrome due to minimal-change disease.
(d) IgA nephropathy.
(e) Acute tubular necrosis.

44. Risk factors for gallstones include:

(a) Iron-deficiency anaemia.
(b) Thyroxine therapy.
(c) Haemolytic anaemia.
(d) Hypoparathyroidism.
(e) Female sex.

45. Regarding diabetes mellitus:

(a) Retinopathy is more likely to be detectable at presentation in late-onset disease than in an adolescent.
(b) Diabetic neuropathy and nephropathy are associated.
(c) Gliclazide causes lactic acidosis in the presence of renal failure.
(d) Insulin is the first-line therapy in a 40-year-old presenting with polyuria, polydipsia, and a raised blood sugar.
(e) Lipohypertrophy is due to poor compliance with diet.

46. Smoking is a risk factor for:

(a) Carcinoma of the bladder.
(b) Parkinson's disease.
(c) Leg ulceration.
(d) Carcinoma of the breast.
(e) Systemic lupus erythematosus.

47. Paget's disease of the nipple is a recognized association with:

(a) Axillary lymphadenopathy.
(b) High-output cardiac failure.
(c) A breast lump.
(d) Hodgkin's disease.
(e) Bloody discharge from the nipple.

48. Myasthenia gravis is associated with:

(a) Abnormal pupil reflexes.
(b) Thymoma.
(c) Anti-acetylcholine antibodies.
(d) Hyperthyroidism.
(e) Double vision.

49. Leg ulcers are associated with:

(a) Turner's syndrome.
(b) Venous insufficiency.
(c) Peripheral neuropathy.
(d) Cryoglobulinaemia.
(e) Bartter's syndrome.

50. In a patient prescribed warfarin:

(a) Aspirin should be prescribed with extreme caution.
(b) If a patient is unable to perform a bleeding time, it should be prescribed with caution.
(c) Binge drinking is potentially dangerous.
(d) Dosage can easily be predicted from the patient's age, sex, and weight.
(e) Patients are advised to take a 'drug holiday' to optimize efficacy.

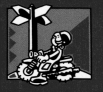

Short-answer Questions

1. What features from the history and examination would suggest the presence of severe aortic stenosis in the presence of an ejection systolic murmur?

2. An elderly patient presents with cough and dyspnoea. What features on physical examination would favour a diagnosis of heart failure?

3. What features on the examination would alert you to a severe attack of asthma?

4. List three of the more common causes of a median nerve palsy at the wrist and describe the physical signs.

5. Describe the features of Parkinson's disease on physical examination.

6. A patient complains of acute lower back pain radiating down the legs. What signs on physical examination would raise the suspicion of an acute disc prolapse of L5–S1?

7. List three causes of massive splenomegaly. Describe the features of a palpable spleen on physical examination.

8. List seven features that may be found on examination of the upper limbs of a patient with long-standing rheumatoid arthritis.

9. List three major causes of papilloedema, and a suggestive feature for each on physical examination.

10. A patient has a breast lump. Describe features on examination that would make you concerned that she has a carcinoma.

11. What mode of transmission is illustrated in Figs 1 and 2? Give two examples of each.

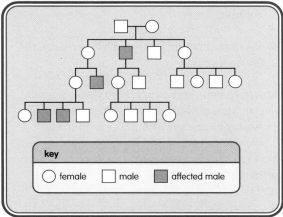

Fig. 1

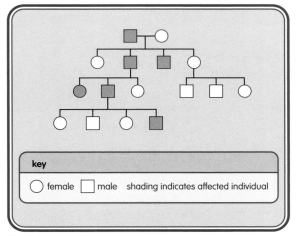

Fig. 2

12. In a patient with acquired immune deficiency syndrome (AIDS), give an example of opportunistic infections that may cause disease in the following:
    (a) Eye.
    (b) Lungs.
    (c) Central nervous system.
    (d) Gastrointestinal tract.
    Give two other groups of patients who may be susceptible to opportunistic infections.

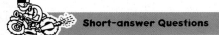

13. A patient presents with anaemia. Give some examples of food that may provide a good dietary source of iron, folate, and vitamin B_{12} to the patient. Give two other examples of causes for each type of anaemia.

14. How may a patient present with hypercalcaemia? Give four causes.

15. A nulliparous woman who is 30 weeks pregnant complains of swollen ankles. What are the three most likely causes? What features on clinical examination would help the differential diagnosis? Which investigations may exclude the more serious causes?

16. List five skin rashes that may be associated with an occult malignancy.

17. Indicate two features in the history and three findings on physical examination that may help to differentiate a hypoglycaemic coma from diabetic ketoacidosis in a diabetic patient.

18. What four questions might you ask a patient with suspected hypothyroidism? Indicate three discriminatory signs that may be present.

19. List four classes of drug that might cause hyperkalaemia and indicate the mechanism.

20. List four risk factors for human immunodeficiency virus (HIV) infection.

1. A 62-year-old man presents with a sudden-onset weakness in his left arm and leg. Discuss how you would assess him in the casualty department and what investigations you would perform.

2. A 30-year-old man is referred to you because his general practitioner hears a systolic murmur during a routine examination. Discuss how your history and examination would guide your further management.

3. An elderly lady has been found by a neighbour lying on the floor. She appeared to be confused and was brought to the local hospital. How would you obtain a history?

4. What features in the history and physical examination would be useful in assessing the long-term control of a 16-year-old boy's asthma?

5. A 45-year-old long-distance lorry driver had been admitted to hospital six weeks earlier with an inferior myocardial infarction. What would you do at his first outpatient assessment following discharge from hospital?

6. A 45-year-old coalminer presents with clubbing. What features on the history and physical examination might elucidate the cause?

7. A 20-year-old man presents with a dry cough, fever, and dyspnoea. What questions would you ask him?

8. An obese 45-year-old lady presents with polyuria and polydipsia. Urinalysis reveals 4+ glucose. What features are important in the history and examination?

9. A 70-year-old man presents to hospital with shortness of breath and marked swelling of his legs. What would you ask him? How would your physical examination help the assessment and what investigations would be most useful in the casualty department?

10. A 20-year-old man reports blood in his urine one week after suffering from a sore throat. What features of the history and examination would guide your further management?

1. (a)F, (b)T, (c)T, (d)T, (e)F

1. (a)F, (b)F, (c)T, (d)F, (e)F   26. (a)T, (b)F, (c)T, (d)F, (e)F

2. (a)F, (b)T, (c)T, (d)F, (e)T   27. (a)F, (b)T, (c)T, (d)T, (e)F

3. (a)T, (b)F, (c)F, (d)F, (e)F   28. (a)T, (b)T, (c)T, (d)T, (e)T

4. (a)F, (b)F, (c)T, (d)T, (e)T   29. (a)T, (b)T, (c)T, (d)F, (e)T

5. (a)F, (b)F, (c)T, (d)T, (e)T   30. (a)T, (b)T, (c)F, (d)T, (e)T

6. (a)T, (b)T, (c)F, (d)T, (e)T   31. (a)F, (b)T, (c)T, (d)F, (e)T

7. (a)T, (b)T, (c)T, (d)T, (e)F   32. (a)F, (b)F, (c)T, (d)T, (e)F

8. (a)T, (b)F, (c)T, (d)F, (e)T   33. (a)T, (b)F, (c)F, (d)F, (e)T

9. (a)T, (b)T, (c)F, (d)T, (e)T   34. (a)T, (b)F, (c)T, (d)F, (e)T

10. (a)F, (b)T, (c)T, (d)F, (e)T   35. (a)F, (b)F, (c)T, (d)T, (e)T

11. (a)T, (b)F, (c)T, (d)F, (e)T   36. (a)F, (b)F, (c)F, (d)T, (e)T

12. (a)F, (b)F, (c)T, (d)F, (e)T   37. (a)F, (b)T, (c)F, (d)T, (e)F

13. (a)T, (b)T, (c)F, (d)F, (e)T   38. (a)T, (b)T, (c)T, (d)F, (e)T

14. (a)F, (b)T, (c)T, (d)F, (e)F   39. (a)F, (b)F, (c)F, (d)T, (e)T

15. (a)T, (b)F, (c)T, (d)F, (e)T   40. (a)F, (b)T, (c)F, (d)T, (e)F

16. (a)F, (b)T, (c)T, (d)F, (e)T   41. (a)F, (b)T, (c)T, (d)F, (e)F

17. (a)T, (b)F, (c)T, (d)T, (e)T   42. (a)T, (b)T, (c)T, (d)T, (e)T

18. (a)T, (b)F, (c)T, (d)F, (e)T   43. (a)F, (b)T, (c)F, (d)T, (e)F

19. (a)T, (b)T, (c)T, (d)F, (e)T   44. (a)F, (b)F, (c)T, (d)F, (e)T

20. (a)T, (b)T, (c)F, (d)T, (e)F   45. (a)T, (b)T, (c)F, (d)F, (e)F

21. (a)T, (b)F, (c)F, (d)F, (e)T   46. (a)T, (b)F, (c)T, (d)F, (e)F

22. (a)F, (b)F, (c)F, (d)T, (e)T   47. (a)T, (b)F, (c)T, (d)F, (e)T

23. (a)T, (b)T, (c)F, (d)T, (e)T   48. (a)F, (b)F, (c)F, (d)T, (e)T

24. (a)T, (b)T, (c)T, (d)F, (e)T   49. (a)F, (b)T, (c)T, (d)T, (e)F

25. (a)F, (b)T, (c)T, (d)T, (e)T   50. (a)T, (b)F, (c)T, (d)F, (e)F

SAQ Answers

1. Features in the history include the triad of :
   - Syncope.
   - Breathlessness on exertion.
   - Angina pectoris.

   Eventually orthopnoea or paroxysmal nocturnal dyspnoea may develop. Features of severe aortic stenosis on examination include:
   - Narrow pulse pressure when recording the blood pressure (e.g. 90/70 mmHg).
   - A slow-rising pulse—small in volume, rises slowly to its peak, and takes a long time to pass the finger.
   - A sustained apex beat suggestive of left ventricular hypertrophy.

2. Features of heart failure include:
   - A displaced apex beat (due to left ventricular volume overload).
   - A third heart sound.
   - An elevated jugular venous pressure.
   - Peripheral oedema.

3. Features of a severe attack of asthma include:
   - Tachycardia (heart rate greater than 110/min).
   - Tachypnoea (respiratory rate greater than 30/min).

- Pulsus paradoxus greater than 15 mmHg.
- Peak expiratory flow rate less than 50% predicted maximum for height and weight.
- Exhaustion.
- Cyanosis.
- Silent chest.
- Bradycardia.
- Difficulty in speaking.

4. Median nerve palsy at the wrist is due to carpal tunnel syndrome. The more common causes include:
   - Pregnancy.
   - Oral contraceptive pill.
   - Hypothyroidism.
   - Rheumatoid arthritis.

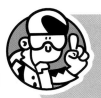

The physical signs include:
- Wasting of the thenar eminence (if long-standing).
- Sensory loss over the palmar aspects of the radial three and a half digits.
- Weakness of abduction, flexion, and opposition of the thumb.
- Tinel's sign—tingling sensation produced in the distribution of the median nerve by percussion over the carpal tunnel.
- Phalen's sign—on flexing the wrists for 60 seconds there is an exacerbation of the paraesthesia, which is rapidly relieved when the wrist is extended.

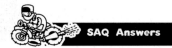

5. The main features of Parkinson's disease are:
   - Tremor (resting, pill-rolling tremor).
   - Bradykinesia.
   - Rigidity ('cog-wheel').

   Other features include an expressionless unblinking face, low-volume monotonous speech, drooling from the mouth, and micrographia. Patients have a characteristic stooping shuffling gait, holding their arms by their side.

6. The signs of an acute disc prolapse may include features of compression of the sciatic nerve roots. Straight leg raising will be impaired on one or both sides—ask the patient to lie flat and lift the leg by the ankle with the knee extended. This will reproduce pain going down the back of the leg. There may be:
   - Sensory loss over the back of the calf and sole of the foot.
   - Weakness of dorsiflexion of the foot.
   - A reduced ankle reflex.

7. Causes of massive splenomegaly include:
   - Chronic myeloid leukaemia.
   - Myelofibrosis.
   - Chronic malaria.

   Features of a palpable spleen on physical examination are:
   - Location in the left upper quadrant of the abdomen.
   - Movement towards the right lower quadrant on inspiration.
   - Dullness to percussion.
   - There may be a notch on the anterior surface.
   - It is not possible to get above the mass.
   - Firm consistency.
   - It cannot be felt bimanually.

8. Any of the following would be acceptable:
   - Symmetrical distribution of joint disease with redness, swelling, warmth, and tenderness.
   - Predominant inflammation in the proximal interphalangeal and metacarpophalangeal joints with relative sparing of the distal interphalangeal joints.
   - Signs of carpal tunnel syndrome.
   - Rheumatoid nodules behind the elbows.
   - Wasting of the small muscles of the hand.
   - Ulnar deviation of the fingers.
   - Deformity of the fingers (e.g. swan neck deformity, boutonnière deformity).

9. The three most common causes of papilloedema are:
   - Intracranial space-occupying lesion.
   - Malignant hypertension.
   - Benign intracranial hypertension.

   Features of these causes include a focal neurological deficit, very high blood pressure, and obesity, respectively.

10. Disturbing features on examination can be divided into local and systemic. Local features include:
    - Mass fixed to deeper tissues.
    - Mass tethered to the skin.
    - Hard and craggy mass.
    - Peau d'orange.
    - Inverted nipple.
    - Associated axillary lymphadenopathy.

    Systemic features include:
    - Hepatomegaly.
    - Pleural effusion.
    - Local bony tenderness.
    - Ascites.

11. Fig. 1 illustrates X-linked recessive inheritance. Examples include:
    - Colour blindness.
    - Haemophilia A.

    Fig. 2 illustrates autosomal dominant inheritance. Examples include:
    - Adult polycystic kidney disease.
    - Dystrophia myotonica.
    - Hereditary spherocytosis.
    - Neurofibromatosis.

12. (a) Cytomegalovirus.
    (b) *Pneumocystis carinii, Mycobacterium avium intracellulare,* cytomegalovirus.
    (c) *Toxoplasma gondii, Cryptococcus neoformans.*
    (d) *Cryptosporidium.*

    Other groups of patients who are at risk of opportunistic infection include transplant recipients who have received immunosuppression and patients receiving chemotherapy or cytotoxic drugs.

13. Iron is found in most meat. This is why vegans are susceptible to iron-deficiency anaemia. Deficiency may also result from chronic blood loss (e.g. menorrhagia, hookworm) or malabsorption (e.g. gastrectomy, coeliac disease).

    Folate is found in most foodstuffs, especially liver, green vegetables, and yeast. Deficiency may also arise from malabsorption (e.g. in coeliac disease, Crohn's disease) or excess use (e.g. due to pregnancy, psoriasis).

    Vitamin B_{12} is found in foods of animal origin only such as liver, fish, and dairy produce. Deficiency may also result from pernicious anaemia, or malabsorption in the ileum (e.g. in Crohn's disease).

14. Hypercalcaemia may present non-specifically or with effect on end-organ damage. The principal sites of presentation include:
    - Kidney—renal stones can cause renal colic, hypercalciuria can cause polyuria and consequent polydipsia.
    - Nervous system—depression, anorexia, nausea and vomiting are common.
    - Gastrointestinal tract—abdominal pain and constipation are commonly associated with hypercalcaemia.
    - Bones—aches and pains.

    Four causes of hypercalcaemia include:
    - Hyperparathyroidism (primary or tertiary).
    - Malignant disease of the bone.
    - Vitamin D excess (e.g. sarcoidosis, iatrogenic).
    - Milk–alkali syndrome.

15. The most likely causes are:
    - Impaired venous drainage of the legs due to the enlarged uterus.
    - Pre-eclampsia.
    - Deep vein thrombosis (increased incidence in pregnancy).

    Discriminatory features on bedside examination would include blood pressure check (hypertension), signs of periorbital oedema, and urinalysis for proteinuria to exclude pre-eclampsia. Features of inflammation such as redness, warmth, and tenderness of the leg would make a deep vein thrombosis more likely.

    Pre-eclampsia may be suggested by the results of a full blood count (thrombocytopenia) urate (raised in pre-eclampsia) and urea and electrolyte estimate (evidence of renal dysfunction). A Doppler ultrasound scan of the leg veins can be performed to look for a deep vein thrombosis. Venography should be avoided if possible in order to minimise the radiation exposure to the fetus.

16. The list is almost endless, but some of the more characteristic signs include:
    - Acanthosis nigricans (especially with gastrointestinal tract malignancy).
    - Dermatomyositis (heliotropic rash).
    - Herpes zoster.
    - Erythema gyratum repens (carcinoma of the breast).
    - Acquired ichthyosis (especially lymphoma).
    - Tylosis (thickening of the palms or soles associated with upper gastrointestinal malignancy).
    - Thrombophlebitis migrans (especially carcinoma of the pancreas).

17. Features in the history include:
    - A defined precipitating cause for diabetic ketoacidosis (e.g. infection, missed an insulin injection) or for hypoglycaemia (e.g. known overdosage of hypoglycaemic treatment or missing a meal).
    - Time course—ketoacidosis usually develops over hours or days, hypoglycaemia is usually associated with a shorter history of illness.

    Features on examination include:
    - Dehydration in patients with ketosis. Patients with hypoglycaemia are usually euvolaemic.
    - Kussmaul's breathing (deep sighing breathing due to acidosis) in ketosis.
    - Sweating (often profound) in a patient with hypoglycaemia.

18. Some questions to ask a patient with suspected hypothyroidism include:
    - "Do you feel more comfortable in warm or cool weather?" to reveal cold intolerance.
    - "Has your weight changed over the past six months?" to reveal weight gain.
    - "Do you have more or less energy now than you used to?" to reveal tiredness, malaise.
    - "Has anyone noticed a change in your facial appearance?"

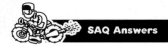

The most discriminatory signs are:
- Bradycardia.
- Slow-relaxing reflexes—easily demonstrated with the ankle reflex.
- Facial appearance (e.g dry coarse hair, periorbital swelling, thinning of eyebrows).

19. Drugs causing hyperkalaemia include:
- Potassium supplements given in excess—cause increased gastrointestinal absorption of potassium.
- Potassium-sparing diuretics (e.g. spironolactone, amiloride)—these drugs antagonize the effect of aldosterone on the distal tubule sodium–potassium exchange pump, resulting in decreased excretion of potassium into the urine.
- Angiotensin-converting enzyme (ACE) inhibitors— decreased angiotensin results in decreased

aldosterone and therefore decreased urinary loss of potassium.
- Nephrotoxic drugs—for example non-steroidal anti-inflammatory drugs (NSAIDs) and aminoglycosides—may cause hyperkalaemia through impaired renal excretion of potassium.

20. Any of the following would be acceptable.
- Haemophilia.
- Blood transfusion in Africa since 1977.
- Sexual partner of a prostitute.
- Intravenous drug user.
- Anal intercourse.
- Multiple sexual partners and unprotected sexual intercourse.
- Sexual partner of an individual in any one of the above groups.

Index

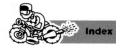

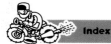

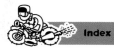

E

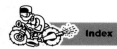

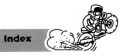

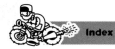

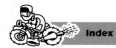

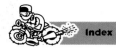

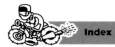

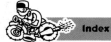

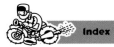